BEYOND DISNEY
Heart of
Healthcare
Excellence

RESTORING THE ART OF COMPASSION AND EMPATHY

by **Fred Lee**
& **Rosemary DeAngelis Laird, MD**

SECOND RIVER
HEALTHCARE

BEYOND DISNEY: Heartwiring Healthcare Excellence

By Fred M. Lee, MA & Rosemary DeAngelis Laird, MD, MHSA

Second River Healthcare
A Healthcare Leadership Publishing Company
26 Shawnee Way, Suite C
Bozeman, MT 59715
FAX (406) 586-5672
Phone (406) 586-8775

Copyright © 2020 Fred M. Lee, MA & Rosemary DeAngelis Laird, MD, MHSA
Editor: Tiffany L. Young
Publisher: Jerry F. Pogue
Cover Design: Megan Marquez
Typesetting/Composition: Neuhaus/Tyrrell Graphic Design
Editing Style: The Chicago Manual of Style – Sixteenth Edition

All rights reserved. No part of this book may be reproduced in any form or by any electronic or mechanical means, or the facilitation thereof, including information storage and retrieval systems, without permission in writing from the publisher, except by a reviewer, who may quote brief passages in a review. Any members of educational institutions wishing to photocopy part or all of the work for classroom use, or publishers who would like to obtain permission to include the work in an anthology, should send their inquiries to Second River Healthcare, 26 Shawnee Way, Suite C, Bozeman, MT 59715

Lee, Fred M. & Laird, Rosemary DeAngelis
Beyond Disney: Heartwiring Healthcare Excellence — Restoring the Art of Compassion and Empathy / Fred M. Lee, MA & Rosemary DeAngelis Laird, MD, MHSA

ISBN-13: 978-1-936406-37-1 (hardcover)
ISBN-13: 978-1-936406-38-8 (softcover)
ISBN-13: 978-1-936406-39-5 (e-book)

1. Healthcare Quality Improvement   2. Compassion and Empathy
3. Patient Experience   4. Patient-Centered Care

Library of Congress Control Number: 2015961034

First Printing   May 2020

Walt Disney Company Trademarks: *Beyond Disney: Heartwiring Healthcare Excellence* is in no way authorized by, endorsed by, or affiliated with the Walt Disney Company, Inc., or Walt Disney World. The Magic Kingdom and Walt Disney World are registered trademarks of the Walt Disney Company. Other Disney trademarks include, but are not limited to, Disneyland, Epcot Center, and Walt Disney. All references to such trademarked properties are used in accordance with the Fair Use Doctrine and are not meant to imply that this book is a Disney product for advertising or other commercial purposes.

Disclaimer: While every precaution has been taken in preparation of this book, the publisher and authors assume no responsibility for errors or omissions. Neither is any liability assumed for damages resulting, or alleged to result, directly or indirectly from the use of the information contained herein. If you do not wish to be bound by the above, you may return this book with receipt to the publisher for a full refund.

Innovative Health Speakers, a speaker's bureau and division of Second River Healthcare, provides a wide range of authors and nationally recognized experts for speaking events. To find out more, go to: **www.InnovativeHealthcareSpeakers.com** or call (406) 586-8775.

Second River Healthcare books are available at special quantity discounts. Please call for information: (406) 586-8775 or order from either website:
www.SecondRiverHealthcare.com

DEDICATION

FROM FRED LEE (1939 – 2017)

To Aura, my wife, best friend, travel agent, and most trusted advisor. Her encouragement kept me motivated after the printing of *If Disney Ran Your Hospital* was published in 2004, and her support allowed me to pursue a passion for speaking and teaching as we traveled around the world and throughout the United States sharing the message of changing one's culture. Her talent as a caregiver, her leadership style as a director of nurses, and her compassion and empathy provided the inspiration and role model for the management principle in *If Disney Ran Your Hospital* and, in this book, *Heartwiring Healthcare Excellence*.

FROM ROSEMARY DeANGELIS LAIRD, MD

Fred and his singularly insightful *9½ Things* inspired many teams of healthcare professionals, family caregivers, and institutions to do better by the patients they serve. Each made courtesy more important than efficiency, continuously worked to improve, and harnessed the motivating power of imagination to close the gap between knowing and doing.

Fred was never more alive than when he relayed to me a visit to a healthcare system or an email from a reader detailing the lessons learned and improvements begun as a result of their reading and implementing the lessons of *If Disney Ran Your Hospital*. I do not think it an overstatement to say Fred felt a duty to complete this book with its message of sustaining the first 9½ *Things*.

To everyone who embraced Fred's message and inspired him to begin *this* book, I dedicate it to you.

Caring for others is a uniquely demanding vocation. Healthcare professionals require highly honed clinical skills and the ability to quickly forge a relationship of respect and trust between themselves and their patients. Fred believed *Heartwiring* is the most important *thing*. I have come to believe it as well.

TABLE OF CONTENTS

Dedication iii

From the Publisher vii

Praise for *Heartwiring Healthcare Excellence* xv

Foreword xxiii

Preface xxix

Introduction xxxvii

SECTION I   Why Healthcare Needs to be *Heartwired* 1

    Chapter 1   A Journey to Healthcare Service Excellence 3

    Chapter 2   Total Quality Management for Healthcare 17

    Chapter 3   The Patient's Story: Judy's Story and the Legend of Gentle Sherry 25

    Chapter 4   Close the Gap Between Knowing and Doing 37

SECTION II   How to *Heartwire* Healthcare 45

    Chapter 5   The Science that Led to a New Era of Medicine .. 49

    Chapter 6   Take Two Placebos and Call Me in the Morning .. 57

    Chapter 7   Compassion + Empathy = *Heartwired* 67

    Chapter 8   Once Upon a Time: The Power of Story 99

**SECTION III The Return on Investment (ROI)
of *Heartwiring*** 111

    Chapter 9   *Heartwiring* for the Win-Win-Win 115

    Chapter 10 Save the Staff: Reduce Burnout and Return
the Joy 131

Conclusion 141

Heartwiring Toolkit 149

About the Authors 167

Glossary 171

Endnotes 175

FROM THE PUBLISHER

I have known Fred Lee since I was in the first grade. We attended Far Eastern Academy together, a small 1st-12th grade school in Singapore operated for children of missionaries located throughout Asia. Fred was a few years older than me. Since it was a small school, the older students watched over the younger ones on school outings. Fred was one of our heroes. He was our "Renaissance Man" before I knew what the meaning of the term was. Suave, debonair, confident, and sophisticated, he had grown up in China, spoke fluent Mandarin Chinese, had lived in Taiwan and Hong Kong, and was someone for a youngster like me to admire. I never stopped looking up to him.

Years later, Fred and I connected again when our mothers lived in the same retirement center. Fred had gone on to work as a Senior Vice President at Florida Hospital in Orlando, one of the largest hospitals in the United States, and then had worked as a cast member at Disney University. Disney recruited him because of his expertise in helping hospitals achieve a culture that inspires patient and employee loyalty. At Disney, he helped adapt and facilitate Disney's Approach to Quality Service and developed a new seminar on Customer Loyalty. I was, by now, part-owner of a healthcare trustee education company and needed a speaker to give a workshop on corporate culture, patient satisfaction, and patient loyalty. Combining our expertise, I asked Fred if he would like to present. He gladly accepted, and it became the first of many workshops hosted by Fred.

To generate more interest in the area, I told Fred to "write a book." After seeing his presentations, I knew he'd be a natural voice of authority with his unique vantage point combining theme parks and hospital wards. Fred went home to Florida and within a few short months delivered seven copies of an excellent manuscript for me to pass along to the major publishing houses. Sadly, *If Disney Ran Your Hospital: 10 Things You Would Do Differently*, was of no interest to any of them. But with Fred on the team, such rejection did not stop us.

Long before self-publishing was a common path to publication, with Fred's book ready to go, I decided to set up a publishing company. I named it Second River Healthcare, A Healthcare Leadership Publishing Company. There was mainstream healthcare, and then there was the alternative, that second river. We wanted to be that alternative publishing company, that would take a fresh look at what healthcare needed to change and improve. We started the publishing company and printed *If Disney Ran Your Hospital* as our first book. By that time, we'd received a valuable recommendation from a college classmate of Fred's, a book editor, who felt the first chapter was only "½ a thing." So, now you know how *If Disney Ran Your Hospital: 9½ Things You Would Do Differently* came to be.

Published in April of 2004, it was named the American College of Healthcare Executives 2005 James A. Hamilton Book of the Year. That first printing sold out in a matter of months and continued to sell. The book is now in five languages: English, Dutch, Portuguese, Korean, and Chinese. We have sold over 500,000 copies worldwide and are in the eighteenth printing as of the date of this book's publication.

When the Chinese licensee heard of Fred's background with China, they asked if he would write a Prologue for the Chinese edition. They said that Chinese readers would be very interested in knowing where Fred's family had lived in China and where Fred had grown up. They were also intrigued by two paragraphs in the introduction to *If Disney Ran Your Hospital* where it stated:

> "In *If Disney Ran Your Hospital*, I am comparing two different corporate cultures in which I have lived and worked. Someone has said, 'He who knows only one culture knows none.'"
>
> "Constantly comparing cultures comes as naturally to me as shaking hands or bowing graciously to a guest. I am the product of two very different cultures. My American parents were both born in China of career missionaries. They lived their whole

lives, except for college and retirement, in China, where I was also born and raised. The infusion of Eastern and Western views on life, work, and family has been as effortless as learning to speak and think in two different languages as a child."

So, Fred lived a personal and professional life at the intersection of two cultures. His unique ability to observe and understand people at their core, not complicated by circumstance or culture, coupled with his storyteller's warmth and charm, placed him at an educator's sweet spot. We have all learned much from him.

After writing *If Disney Ran Your Hospital* and winning the ACHE 2005 Book of the Year, glowing reviews followed in major healthcare journals, and sales took off. Speaking appointments poured in, changing Fred and Aura's life forever, after translations in several languages (including most recently in Fred's beloved Chinese), the book became one of the best-selling books in healthcare history.

FRED'S SECOND BOOK

Since his first book, Fred began the dream for a second. He didn't want it to be a sequel but wanted something new with original research. He was working on the manuscript and sending me chapters as he completed them when I received the following.

········· UNEXPECTED BULLETIN! ·········

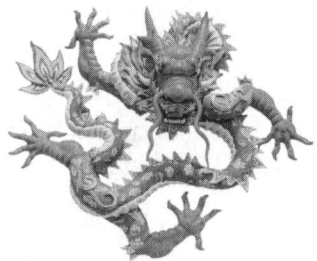

It matters little in the end, whether I slew the dragon, or he devoured me, only that I stared him down smiling.

~ Fred Lee, 2016

As if fate conspired to give me a lesson in procrastination, a malevolent dragon called GBM-4 found a lair on the surface of my brain, placing me under the spell of a death sentence.

After two years of research for the content, I had begun to put together the themes and some chapters of this book. Then my 46-year-old son died from an insulin reaction in October 2014. Six months later, I began to deteriorate physically–low energy. No appetite. I wanted to sleep all the time. The book seemed like a millstone around my neck.

I went to my primary care physician, Monisha Seth. She ran some tests. (Low Vitamin B-12. Low Vitamin D. Borderline low testosterone) It looked like I might be having some weakness on my left side. Better include a cardiologist, hematologist, and a neurologist to be safe. The cardiology stress test was good. Hematology report normal. Growing consensus: Grief over the death of my son.

However, Dr. Slansky, the neurologist did a vigorous exam and thought he detected a slight drifting in my left hand. "It could be a very small stroke," he said. "We need an MRI. Where do you want to go?" We weren't sure. "There is a place up the street where I can order one STAT and get a report immediately," he said. We agreed.

After the first pass through the MRI, the radiologist came out of her office and said, "There is something there. It's either a bleed or a mass. We need to take some more pictures. It should take fifteen minutes."

I said, "Could you get my wife, Aura Lee, from the waiting room?" Aura was able to stand beside me. Under the brace that held my head in place, someone had put a small mirror beside my face so we could maintain eye contact throughout the test.

After another short wait, the radiologist returned. "It's a mass," she said. "We have told your neurologist, and he has already sent orders for you to be admitted to the hospital through the emergency department immediately." "Can you go right now?" "Yes, of course, we can go now," we said with an anxious look into each other's eyes and a blurry hug as frightened tears began to well.

And so, life can show you in a split second how fragile and vulnerable we all are, and how quickly the ground can shift under our feet. Of course, we all know this, and it has happened to millions of people before us. But surely no one is ever ready for it when it does. For us, it was like being blindsided by a sucker punch.

The day was Aura's birthday. Luckily the neurosurgeon, Ravi Gandhi, was on call and specialized in brain tumors. He was excited about a new technique that used a chemical that lit up the tumor cells in fluorescent green dye. I signed the papers for it, and he assured us that he could remove 90-95 percent of the tumor. The surgery took five hours. He announced that he had gotten 100 percent of the fluorescent cells. So I was admitted to Florida Hospital's Neuro ICU on Wednesday, surgery on Friday, and discharged on Sunday afternoon!

We waited for the pathology report. During the follow-up visit with Dr. Slansky, he asked if we wanted to hear the pathology report or wait for the surgeon to tell us. I said, "Shoot, the sooner, the better." The words and phrases exploded like bombs.

Glioblastoma
Stage 4 most advanced stage
Most malignant
100 percent reoccurring
Life expectancy for a man your age 12-18 months

"What's in store for you now," Dr. Slansky continued, "is lots of MRIs and maybe PET scans under the supervision of your neuro-oncologist, to keep a close watch on any reoccurrence."

After thinking it all over, I said, "So your vigorous neuro exam saved my life." He said, "Well, what really saved your life is that you noticed something was wrong, told your family, and they got you in here right away. You are the fastest diagnosis, surgery, and post-op I have ever had! Really quite amazing."

So, surprisingly, I am energized, focused, optimistic, and abundantly hopeful. My brain seems to have been rebooted with my college brain. Words come easier, files more accessible, memory doubled (although my surgeon says it's the steroids!) My mantra has become, "My cup runs over, but there's no time to lollygag." And one more:

"Depend upon it, sir, when a man knows he is to be hanged in a fortnight, it concentrates his mind wonderfully."
~ Samuel Johnson

MEETING ROSEMARY deANGELIS LAIRD, MD

While Fred was fighting his Stage Four Glioblastoma, I was visiting him at his home in Florida, where I met one of his physicians, Rosemary DeAngelis Laird, MD. Dr. Laird had become the Executive Medical Director of the AdventHealth Senior Health and concurrently founded the Centre for Senior Health at AdventHealth Winter Park Hospital. Dr. Laird and Fred had a connection. They both believed in compassionate and empathetic care. She had been a fan of Fred's years earlier after reading his first book, *If Disney Ran Your Hospital*. Dr. Laird had some experience in book writing. She co-authored the 2009 Best Consumer Health Book titled: *Take Your Oxygen First: Protecting Your Health and Happiness While Caring for a Loved One with Memory Loss*.

Dr. Laird is a Fellow of the American Geriatrics Society and received the American Geriatrics Society Clinician of the Year award in 2013. After many discussions between Fred and Dr. Laird, Fred asked her if she would facilitate his transferring his extensive library to AdventHealth University, (formerly Adventist University of Health Sciences) founded by AdventHealth Orlando (formerly Florida Hospital). Dr. Laird facilitated that request, and now Fred's vast collection of books and many of his notes called the "Fred Lee Special Collection" reside at the R. A. Williams Library at AdventHealth University in Orlando.

After his passing, Fred's wife, Aura, Dr. Laird, and I talked about having Dr. Laird finish *Heartwiring*, which Fred had been working on before and during his illness. With that agreement, we began pulling all of Fred's research and work together for Dr. Laird to bring to you the culmination of their book, *Heartwiring Healthcare Excellence.*

Dr. Laird has been working diligently on this book while operating a busy program at AdventHealth. She has gone above and beyond all expectations.

We offer you this book, which has been a great collaboration between Fred Lee, the administrator, and Rosemary DeAngelis Laird, MD, the physician. Yet another crucial cross-cultural combination! I believe my great friend Fred would be pleased.

Fred passed away on Sunday evening, March 26, 2017, with his family gathered around him.

Jerry F. Pogue,
Publisher

PRAISE FOR
HEARTWIRING
HEALTHCARE EXCELLENCE

When we hired Fred Lee at Disney, it was to bring his healthcare perspective to our new program on delivering world-class service. Working with Fred was a life-changing experience. His insights have proven to be transformative to the healthcare industry, and I'm thrilled to see his continued thought leadership throughout Beyond Disney: Heartwiring Healthcare Excellence, written with Dr. Rosemary Laird. This new content is a long- overdue game-changer! Every healthcare leader who desires better patient outcomes and staff engagement should share these valuable insights on how to provide the most effective, compassionate care... and optimize the potential of your hospital!

Mark David Jones
Former Disney Executive
President of Small World Alliance, Inc.
Orlando, Florida

In my work with hospitals, I have long pointed out that research shows that the better the patient experience, the better the health outcomes. In Heartwiring Healthcare Excellence, the late, great Fred Lee and

Dr. Rosemary DeAngelis Laird show why: the relationship that patients have with their providers—with every human being they encounter while under care—is a core part of the therapeutic process. Read this book fervently, thoroughly, and closely to Heartwire your experience.

B. Joseph Pine II
Co-Author, The Experience Economy
Co-Founder, Strategic Horizons
Dellwood, Minnesota

....

Fred Lee and Rosemary DeAngelis Laird, MD, have written another unforgettable, thought provoking masterpiece, following Lee's highly acclaimed If Disney Ran Your Hospital: 9½ Things You Would Do Differently *(2004). This time they focused on making empathetic care 'heartwired' into every process, system, and person who works in healthcare. How to sustain compassion when you are tired and at the end of your 12-hour shift? How to design better healthcare systems and processes that help us recharge our emotional energies to continue to offer that smile—the ultimate placebo that all humans can give to another? Find out about the four strategies to transform your team from 'talking the talk' to 'walking the walk'.*

There is so much to take away from this book: strategies and tactical plans for heartwiring compassionate, personalized care in individuals and in your organization, memorable quotes that will be used in presentation slide decks, human stories to share and reflect, how Schwartz Rounds, PDSA cycles, and TQM (Total Quality Management) all work alongside narrative medicine to provide more compassionate care for patients. I particularly love the Daisy Story describing a motivating exercise we can all do with our team in order to put ourselves in someone else's shoes and the Stone Mason story for finding staff with more positive attitude.

This book is invaluable for all healthcare workers and carers who wish to continue to deliver high-quality patient care with big hearts. It is equally indispensable to all industries and business leaders who are looking to create a more personalized customer interaction that will generate great memories and stories that your customers will share for years to come.

Sue Kong, MBA, MSc, Chartered Marketer (CIM)
Director
National Health Service (NHS) – Elect
London, United Kingdom

In times of budget- and regulation-driven healthcare, it is absolutely inspiring to read Heartwiring Healthcare Excellence: Restoring the Art of Compassion and Empathy, *in which Fred Lee and Dr. Rosemary DeAngelis Laird guide us from hardwired healthcare to the concept of Heartwiring: The inclusion of Compassion plus Empathy into our patient-focused care, resulting in true caring, without losing sight of economic drivers.*

While the authors provide robust scientific substantiation on everything they state, the book still reads like a page-turner.

A true masterpiece and a must-read for all involved in the care of fellow human beings.

Jaap Verweij, MD, PhD
Dean of the Faculty of Medicine (Retired)
Vice-Chairman of the Board of Directors (Retired)
Erasmus University Medical Center
Rotterdam, Netherlands

Fred Lee was one of a kind: A world renowned author and speaker and—as is the fate of most of us—eventually, a patient. Fred filled a room with his presence and shared his passion for the patient experience with countless readers for decades. Fred's message was simple, it was contagious, and it was an inspiration. He wanted **every** healthcare worker to look at our actions, our words, and our culture through the patient perspective. But this latest book, written with Dr. Rosemary DeAngelis Laird, goes further to challenge all of us to not only hardwire to get results but also "heartwire" our healthcare excellence by restoring the art of compassion and empathy.

I'm not surprised that Fred worked until the end of his life trying to make a difference for all of us by writing another book. Driving home the fact that quality care is not just about outcomes but also about how well we care **about and with** our patients. I'm also not surprised that he was able to pen this book with his own physician, Dr. Laird. Their book provides us insight into the power of how caregiver compassion and empathy can impact a patient mindset, decrease their fears, affect their outcomes, and hopefully help us remember the **WHY** of our work... our patient.

During these times in our world filled with fear and unknown, there is no better time for those of us in healthcare to slow down and create connections with our patients; anticipate their fears and help them feel safe. I can only imagine that the pride and joy that is generated in us as we provide compassion and empathy to our patients creates a win-win, possibly even preventing provider burnout. Thank you, Fred, for your mentorship and the legacy you left behind and Rosemary for carrying on that legacy of compassion and empathy.

Katie Lydon MSN, RN, NE-BC, CPXP
Director, Women and Children's Services
NorthBay Healthcare
NorthBay Healthcare Hospitals, Magnet Recognized®
Fairfield, California

The greatest thing a man can do is to leave a legacy of change, as Mother Teresa said, "I alone cannot change the world, but I can cast a stone across the waters to create many ripples." In Fred's final treatise, Beyond Disney: Heartwiring Healthcare Excellence *with Dr. Rosemary DeAngelis Laird, they are creating a tsunami effect of Heart transplants and is the antidote to a stressed world and healthcare system. And as a gesture of paying it forward, Dr. Laird gives everybody, from the individual through the manager up to the C-Suite executive, the "Heartwiring Toolkit" to make the transplant easier. This book is the prescription for an ailing system and needs to be read and implemented now!*

Phillip Zinni III, DO, FAOASM, ATC
National Medical Director
THE INDUSTRIAL ATHLETE
Reno, Nevada

Past-President
American Osteopathic Academy of Sports Medicine

....

Fred Lee has certainly planted many seeds around the world in how healthcare providers can take care of patients with compassion and empathy. Gratitude is the word that comes to my mind when I read this book, because his works always touch me and transform me as a professional and as a human being. Lee's concepts reflect the way I aim to work. Therefore, I desire to spread and multiply his experience as an educator. After all, the important thing is to take care of our patients with Heartwiring Healthcare Excellence! *Thank you very much. I´m elated to be part of this small, yet gratifying opportunity that will definitely spread innumerous fertile seeds in the worldwide.*

Regina Kaneko, RN, M.Sc.
Consultant and Director
SIMSAFETY
Sao Paulo, Brazil

Heartwiring Healthcare Excellence *is a compelling tribute that is the antidote to provider burnout in this age of RVU-based quantification of productivity; is a re-focusing on patient-centered delivery of compassionate and empathetic care and experiencing the human dimension of medicine. Our motivation to create a positive therapeutic experience for the patient* **will** *play a significant role in the positive outcome we provide as healers. In fact, every outcome will be positive if it is heartwired, including end of life.*

David Michael, MD, FACOG
Chief Visionary
North Shore Pediatric Therapy
Des Plaines, Illinois

After Fred Lee's first book, many healthcare professionals opened their eyes for a better quality and outcome of care. Not by complicated management strategies but a patient-friendly, empathetic approach to patients. In addition, Fred had the gift to be a clear communicator transferring knowledge easily from the CEO to the cleaner. His posthumous book Heartwiring Healthcare Excellence *written with Rosemary Laird, MD, is a clear deepening of this subject. Again, an excellently written book with a clear but, above all, simple message for every healthcare professional on how to improve outcome for patients. It shows: A Heartwiring approach is for free, but it becomes priceless when you practice it.*

Robert Slappendel, MD, PhD
Anesthesiologist
Professor Safety and Quality in Healthcare
Tilburg, Netherlands

Fred Lee's If Disney Ran Your Hospital *introduced us to a patient-centric journey for a better patient experience. Fred Lee and Rosemary DeAngelis Laird's new book,* Heartwiring Healthcare Excellence, *takes us further on that journey. To be Heartwired is to know and use the patient's story to provide quality care and to design a healthcare system that restores the art of compassion and empathy. It is another must read for every healthcare leader.*

Tony Bennett
Chief Executive Officer
Encompass Health Rehabilitation Hospital of Panama City
Panama City, Florida

FOREWORD

I still remember the first time I read Fred Lee's *If Disney Ran Your Hospital: 9½ Things You Would Do Differently*. It was 2007. I was stepping into the role of interim CEO of UCLA Health, and thinking about what it meant to deliver care that truly puts patients first. At the time, UCLA was renowned for its world-class physicians–but was ranked in the 38th percentile for patient satisfaction among US hospitals. Something was seriously wrong.

Fred's book resonated with me, reinforcing what I'd learned during my years as a child and adolescent psychiatrist: You have to treat patients like people with real lives, not just case files. You need to provide for the whole person, giving them engaging, compassionate—and yes, even delightful—experiences. Top-notch care alone isn't enough to help people heal and move forward. And when you treat your patients that way, you offer better, more personalized care, as well. Everybody wins.

At UCLA Health, we set about establishing a "one patient at a time" approach and updated our mission statement to focus on "Healing humankind, one patient at a time, by alleviating suffering, promoting health, and delivering acts of kindness." We really lived that mission, too. That's how we rose to the 99th percentile in patient satisfaction, becoming the nation's most-recommended hospital. And we got there by simply shifting our way of thinking; Instead of worrying about the numbers, we said, "Let's do what's right for the patient."

Some of our approach was Disney-esque, but it was the little things we did —things that other hospitals weren't doing—that made the biggest difference. For instance, we introduced ourselves to each patient, and told them what we were doing (and going to do) every step of the way. We explained everything in relatable human, not clinical, terms.

We even huddled our housekeeping staff nightly and shared fun facts, like "Today is the 70th anniversary of Little League." Why? Because we wanted them to go into patient rooms, introduce themselves, and say, "Is there a part of the room you want me to clean that needs special attention? Oh, and by the way, did you know that today is the 70th anniversary of Little League?" Simple facts like that started conversations that fostered meaningful relationships between our staff and patients.

Which is why, when I picked up Fred's book in 2007 just as I was embarking on my transition at UCLA, I realized, "Yeah, this is exactly the same journey that we're on."

Fred began working on the book that you hold in your hands (or in your e-reader) before his death in 2017; it was completed by his exceptional collaborator, Dr. Rosemary DeAngelis Laird. *Beyond Disney: Heartwiring Healthcare Excellence* expands upon the principles in Fred's first book and takes a closer look at the role of compassion, empathy, and the mind-body connection in healing.

The essence of the book is about shifting from our current "hardwired" standard of clinical care to a more human and holistic *"Heartwired"* approach. As noted in the introduction, "To be *Heartwired* is to know and use the patient's story to provide quality care with genuine compassion and empathy." This message—and this book—couldn't come at a more critical time. As we face unprecedented challenges that risk overwhelming our global healthcare systems, it's more important than ever to reflect on how we care for people, not just patients.

The message of *Beyond Disney: Heartwiring Healthcare Excellence* is deceptively simple: By connecting deeply with patients through compassion and empathy, we empower them to heal themselves in partnership with their caregivers. This isn't just about improving customer service or the patient experience—it's about reinventing healthcare so that it's human-centered, driven by compassion, and shaped by our shared experiences on this earth. It's also about how the power of imagination and belief in our innate ability to heal can save lives.

I now write this foreword while leading Google Health, where I have the opportunity to scale the delivery of authoritative information to millions of people and build tools for people to help them live healthier and happier lives. While our impact is driven by the incredible power of technology such as artificial intelligence, the same people-first approach still applies. At Google, respect for the user is our number-one value. That same focus drove the fundamental shift we made at UCLA, and that Fred so eloquently espoused in his first book, and now in his last.

Even as we strive to do the right thing, we can't claim that the job is finished. Because, if we really cared for the whole person, healthcare would be affordable, it would be understandable, it would be accessible. It would be culturally dignified and sensitive, and it would be universal. Everybody should get the right kind of healthcare, not just what's best for the healthcare provider or system. And that's at the heart of this book's message as well: Treat people as human beings (not numbers) and connect. Simply and truly connect.

David T. Feinberg, MD, MBA
Vice President
Google Health
Mountain View, California

Former President & CEO
Geisinger Health System
Danville, Pennsylvania

Former President & CEO
UCLA Health
Los Angeles, California

If Disney Ran Your Hospital You Would…

Redefine your Competition and Focus on What Can't be Measured (This is the ½ Thing)

Make Courtesy More Important than Efficiency

Regard Patient Satisfaction as Fool's Gold

Measure to Improve, Not to Impress

Decentralize the Authority to say YES

Change the Concept of Work from Service to Theater

Harness the Motivating Power of Imagination

Create a Climate of Dissatisfaction

Cease Using Competitive Monetary Rewards to Motivate People

Close the Gap Between Knowing and Doing

PREFACE

What is *Heartwiring*?

What if there was an immune-boosting, pain-reducing, all-purpose drug therapy, rigorously tested and confirmed with hundreds of double-blind clinical trials, which has been shown to improve clinical outcomes in up to 42 percent of hospital patients; cut length of stay after major surgery and wound care by 25 percent; and reduce readmission rates due to poor patient compliance by 60 percent? And what if it has virtually zero negative side effects and can prevent over 70 percent of all medical malpractice lawsuits, while significantly improving patients' overall rating of care? Such therapy exists. In recent years it has achieved increased acceptance among medical experts who once doubted it. In 2011, Harvard University Medical School and its teaching hospital, Beth Israel Deaconess Medical Center, founded an institute to study its processes and specific effects on the neurological, endocrine, and immune systems. Much of this exciting new research was made possible by more advanced brain imaging technology than has ever been available before.

The therapy's name is *placebo*, from the Latin "I shall please." The effects ascribed to it are in part caused by the intangible connection created by the patient-caregiver relationship through *empathy, trust, hope, suggestion, expectation,* and *compassion*. I call it **Heart**wiring in contrast to **hard**wiring because the efficacy of this therapy is wholly dependent on a genuine, personalized heart-to-heart connection between caregivers and their patients.

> We may be able to have excellence in quality metrics without it, but I do not think we can achieve greatness in the healing experience, or staff work life, without it. ~ **Fred Lee**

If you have read *If Disney Ran Your Hospital: 9½ Things You Would Do Differently* and your hospital or healthcare system has embedded these teachings, you are well on your way to being ready for *Beyond Disney: Heartwiring Healthcare Excellence*. If you are new to this series, welcome! A list of the *9½ Things* you will want to do differently is provided on page xxvii, but you will surely benefit from reading the first book as well. After I first read *If Disney Ran Your Hospital*, I was immediately hooked. I found it a uniquely thoughtful offering about the consumer experience in healthcare that was prescient in suggesting the relationship between healthcare provider and a patient is the fundamental driver creating quality and value. This was "patient-centeredness" before anyone had used that term. I was keen to meet the author. As so often happens, however, our path to meeting took some time, twists of fate, and unwelcome turns.

At the time of the book's release in 2004, Fred was invited to speak to the physicians and management teams of my local healthcare system. Unfortunately, I had a conflict and had to miss the presentation. The event was highly lauded, and it created quite an impact across our system for some time. Fast forward several years and I learned about another opportunity to see and hear Fred speak. How many authors are on book tours eleven years after the book is released? *If Disney Ran Your Hospital* and those *9½ Things* aren't just the customer service flavor of the month! I was determined to meet Fred at this next opportunity. I had already read the book of course, but to brush up on it before I heard him speak, I purchased and listened to the audiobook.

For the next ten hours, my commute was pure joy. I replayed parts of the book simply to hear him tell a story. But the *9½ Things* was no mere collection of stories. It is a brilliantly crafted manual of strategies to infuse compassion and empathy within healthcare. Sadly, the event was canceled. At the time we were told, "Mr. Lee is ill and the event would be rescheduled." Disappointment again, but this time I had a plan. I learned he and his wife lived in the central Florida area, so I decided to reach out to him.

From: Rosemary.Laird.MD
To: Fred Lee
Sent: Sunday, September 4, 2016 2:28 AM
Subject: Florida Hospital physician-gratitude and requests

Mr. Lee,

My daily commute this week from Melbourne to Winter Park has been an absolute delight! I've been listening to you present *If Disney Ran Your Hospital*.

Thank you for writing the book. Your explanation of imagination as the source of empathy is genius. And, as a geriatrician, your use of anecdotes involving the care of elders touched and inspired me personally and professionally.

My next reason for writing is more involved. The focus of my work is improving care for seniors across the healthcare system. Would you be willing to partner with me on developing a handbook for healthcare personnel focused on strategies for developing healthcare teams that embody and regularly deliver compassionate, empathetic, and best-practice care for elders?

It would be an absolute honor to speak with you further about these items.

With gratitude and admiration,

Rosemary Laird, MD, MHSA
Geriatrician, Florida Hospital Medical Group

P.S. I thought perhaps you'd be interested in knowing that Dr. Atul Gawande is coming to town as part of the Distinguished Lecture Series sponsored by Florida Hospital. He will be speaking on his book *Being Mortal* Wednesday, September 21st at 6 pm at the Dr. Phillips Center. If you are interested in attending, please let me know and I will obtain tickets for you.

When the reply arrived the next day, I read it with a mix of elation, admiration, and heartbreak.

From: Fred Lee
To: Rosemary.Laird.MD
Sent: Monday, September 5, 2016 7:22 AM
Subject: Florida Hospital physician-gratitude and requests

Dear Dr. Laird:

Your email made my day! If endorphins stimulate the immune system which is important in fighting cancer, then it was positively therapeutic.

Almost exactly a year ago, a neurosurgeon took a stage 4 glioblastoma multiforme (GBM) brain tumor out of my cranium. I was told my life expectancy was 14 months, and it has now been 12 $^1/_2$ months. Tomorrow I get another MRI to see if there is any sign of a recurrence. So you can see why Atul Gawande's *Being Mortal* has been especially valuable to my family and me. Attached is a bookmark I had made up when I got my GBM. You will see that I quote Gawande with a favorite quote on the back side of the bookmark. You will need to scroll down on the image to get the backside. So, *yes*, I do want to hear Gawande speak.

The answer to your question is YES. I'd be happy to collaborate with you on your project. We should try to meet in the next couple of weeks. **I should tell you that I am working feverishly on a second book in what little time I may have left.** In a separate email, I will send you some PowerPoint slides from a talk I sometimes give to long-term care staff. If you are curious to put my voice to a mental picture of me giving a talk, there is a YouTube of me giving a TEDx TALK in the Netherlands here: https://www.youtube.com/watch?v=tylvc9dY400

Fred
Fred Lee & Associates, Inc.

Of course, the next clicks on my computer brought up what is cited as the best video of all time about patient experience. It is a masterful performance and fitting culmination of years of study and collaboration with countless hospital systems and healthcare professionals. Within a few days, my husband (a family medicine physician) and I met Fred and his devoted and wise healthcare muse, his wife Aura. Her lifelong work as a Registered Nurse and Director of Nursing gave Fred many elements of his real-life healthcare experiences to draw on before his own illness brought him the personal exposure he used in his second book. Over the next months, our work continued when his health would allow.

I learned of Fred's extensive work researching the role of the placebo effect. I had my eyes—and mind—opened wide at the science emerging that underscores the bio-psycho-social model of healthcare and patient/clinician interaction. As I learned more about Fred's theory about *Heartwiring*, it seemed a natural progression of his early work. At its core what Fred identified while watching Disney cast members, was what Walt Disney himself identified when he said of his park, "We want people to feel it is the happiest place on Earth." It is the *feeling for the individual* that is the critical contribution from Disney associates. Similarly, while no one would equate a day at Disney to a day in the operating room, and the healthcare provider may have to deliver bad news, it is the *emotional connection* made between the patient and the clinician or other healthcare associates that truly creates the quality in healthcare. Fred found this connection and made it more attainable for all of us.

I was given the unique and humbling opportunity to show my *Heartwiring* to the master himself. As the options for treating Fred's cancer ran out, it became clear the end would be coming soon. Fred and Aura felt I, as a Geriatrician, could understand their wishes for his end-of-life care. I was honored when they asked me to be his physician. So, over the last six months of Fred's life, I filled that role as well. Fortunately, I had some help from another physician whose book, *Being Mortal*, brought new awareness to the importance of patient-centered, end-of-life planning.

In September 2016, not long after Fred and I met, Dr. Atul Gawande came to Orlando as a special guest for a speaking event focusing on *Being Mortal*. Fred had read *Being Mortal* and was eager to meet Dr. Gawande. Fortune smiled on us and the meeting took place. That Dr. Gawande graciously acknowledged and praised *If Disney Ran Your Hospital* meant a great deal to Fred personally and professionally.

In *Being Mortal*, Dr. Gawande speaks to the power of the individual in determining their course of care. In *9½ Things* Fred teaches that respect and compassion for the individual should be a foundational aspect, nurtured, maintained, and supported not only in death, or near death, but always. As his time was drawing near, Fred was becoming a bit unsettled and desperate to finish [t]his book. In one of our last conversations with Fred (my husband and I were with him), we used a strategy described by Dr. Gawande to prioritize his final days. Apart from his family, he identified teaching as "what mattered most" to him. Using an example from *Being Mortal*, we shifted his focus from working on his book to working toward "one final piano recital." Instead, for Fred, it would be "one final lesson." Aura arranged to have former students come and see Fred. Many more than she had ever anticipated came, and it was an immensely gratifying experience for all of them.

In the coming pages, Fred and I teach what he learned through discussions with thousands of readers in the years after *If Disney Ran Your Hospital* was published, and through his personal observations of being a patient after brain cancer was diagnosed. Those 9½ *Things* have touched many personal and professional lives.

After we'd been working together for a bit, Fred mentioned he thought it was helpful that I am a physician. I explained the relatively recent trend toward "dyad leadership" where a physician or other clinician works alongside someone trained in business to make decisions about all aspects of patient care and healthcare delivery. He smiled and said that meant he and Aura were "way ahead of their time!" Indeed, they were.

Fred came to believe, achieving greatness in the healing professions requires a heart wired to care, even more than it requires a mind replete with knowledge or hands with specialized skills. Our ultimate thesis, building on the 9½ *Things*, is that top-decile providers are *Heartwired* with a foundation of compassion and empathy turning knowledge and skills into acts of high-quality care. Curricula will often focus on knowledge, skills, and attitudes but perhaps attitudes should set the stage for what follows and not be in the trailing position.

Fred desperately wanted to teach this final lesson, spending much of his last year completing research and writing several chapters. Born into a missionary family, he was educated broadly and experienced life thoughtfully. From an early age, he identified his gifts to educate and motivate others. Most recently his pupils are healthcare professionals striving for excellence. Fred did much during his life for others. It is fitting that he left lessons that will endure for years far beyond his time on Earth. Here we present his final and, I believe, most impactful lesson. If anyone was *Heartwired*, it was Fred Lee. May your life and work be forever changed as mine has been.

Dr. Rosemary DeAngelis Laird

INTRODUCTION

"A hospital without compassion would be like Disney without fun."
~ Fred Lee

HEARTWIRING HEALTHCARE EXCELLENCE

With the release of *If Disney Ran Your Hospital: 9½ Things You Would Do Differently*, we were ushered into a new era of patient-centric healthcare delivery. Fred's wise and visionary counsel was formed at the unlikely intersection of an emergency room on Main Street, USA. It is somewhat intuitive that one will be happy at the "Happiest Place on Earth," so what could healthcare possibly learn that would leave an ill and broken patient better off, and dare we say it, happy to have been at the hospital? No mere transaction buoyed by "Disney" level customer satisfaction principles, a patient-centric healthcare event should be an interpersonal interaction *Heartwired* with the curative cocktail of compassion and competence present in equal measure.

In Section 1, we begin with an exploration of how healthcare has arrived at the value-based and patient-centered world we are in today, where clinical quality, outcomes, and satisfaction collectively define and drive us. It didn't start out that way. So we will review the evolution of customer service from a marketing tool to key quality, performance, and satisfaction indicators. The shift from thinking of healthcare as a service to an emotional experience was a critical paradigm shift. The standards for performance were held for too long in the service economy model. Worse yet, the important lessons of continuous quality improvement that moved some industries far forward were incompletely applied in healthcare settings. What part is missing? The perspective of the patient. Disney's *pixie dust* is the individualized care and attention paid to the emotional experience of the guest. How can healthcare do the same? How can the emotional experience of a patient be factored into the healthcare encounter? Through patient-centered care.

Every patient is a person who has a story, not a "case" distinguished by a disease. The "gallbladder in 205" is actually Ms. Micelli, the watercolor artist and avid runner, who is both in pain from an as-yet-unidentified complication of her surgery last week and worried about her 10- and 12-year-old children now home alone until their grandmother arrives later tonight. What we learn from a patient's story and the attitude of wanting to know a patient's story, comes together as the *pixie dust* healthcare needs to create the compassionate and empathetic care required in the value-based era. Core competencies for all healthcare providers must now go beyond hardwired service excellence. To be **Heartwired** is to **know and use the patient's story to provide quality care with genuine compassion and empathy**.

Can modern healthcare move from being Hardwired to *Heartwired*? We believe it can. *Heartwiring* a healthcare system with a culture of genuine compassion and empathy creates a healthy and capable workforce able to achieve robust and sustainable outcomes in patient-centered, high-value care. It is the modern necessity for a successful leap from good to great.

In Section 2, we move from theory to action. How can we become *Heartwired* and lead others in that direction as well? First, we explore the basics of human interaction and the origins of a model of interpersonal interaction now well known as the bio-psycho-social model. Groundbreaking in its day, it began the push of clinicians toward more personal rather than solely technical encounters. We will review recent evidence of just how active the mind-body connection is in regulating physical and emotional states. For modern-day healthcare workers who want to perform at their highest level, and clinicians who wish to heal with compassion and promote whole-person health, learning to be *Heartwired* is the key.

As social beings, human interactions have a broad and direct influence over our general well-being and health. *Heartwired* associates will need to carry new skill sets that include the knowledge, skills, and attitudes of promoting healthy mind-body connections. The ability to create a positive therapeutic connection between a healthcare provider and patient can mean the difference between health and disease. Think that's touchy-feely nonsense or want to pass it off as unsubstantiated hogwash? Read on for an updated perspective on mind over matter and a new understanding of placebo.

No longer regarded as underhanded trickery, we have a far more sophisticated understanding of placebo and its potential for altering a physical process. Well beyond its use as a sham pill, researchers have identified that the provider-patient relationship itself is part of the "placebo effect" and through that connection, a unit of change. Beyond the pill or surgery, the relationship takes an active role in therapeutic outcomes. A *Heartwired* provider can be just the therapeutic ally a patient needs. Nurses or therapists can communicate and interact with patients in specific ways to make success more likely. Did you know a smile contains a certain amount of the cure? A patient's positive attitude can reduce stress and allow the immune system to function more effectively. As patients do the work of healing, we can help them by being *Heartwired*.

Next, we will explore the process of *Heartwiring* healthcare associates with a foundation of compassion and empathy to guide and enhance their performance. Is compassion innate or can it be a learned skill? What about empathy? Are some of us born to care more than others? To begin, we define these uniquely valuable but commonly confused attributes and evaluate their role in the patient experience. Then we look at strategies to promote the development of healthcare providers as skilled in compassion and empathy as they are in the specific clinical aspects of their roles.

To further develop clinicians with empathy, we will look to the emerging field of narrative medicine that is illuminating the value contained within key aspects of our patient's story and how such a story influences a patient's experience. Often forgotten in the sterility of medicine is the context of illness within a human story, a human life. Who is this person with pneumonia? Is it a "hot gallbladder" in 430A? No! It is a married 44-year-old university professor and mother of two with her second bout of acute cholecystitis (an acutely painful infection of the gallbladder). What does the patient want? How does this illness affect her, her family? What is she hoping for, fearing, expecting? Along the way, we will meet several patients and hear from administrators working to improve their care. In most cases, throughout the book, we've changed the names to protect privacy, but you will also see we've included the names of patients and healthcare administrators who wanted their story to further this vital message. Knowing and appreciating our patient's story is indeed a necessary tenet of being *Heartwired* and propels us toward more effective points of interaction with our patients.

In Section 3, we come face to face with the elephant in the room. Can we afford to be *Heartwired*? Compassion and empathy sound good, but will they support the margin and allow the mission? Sure, an employee at Disney can spend time ensuring satisfaction among their happy vacationers, but this is healthcare where sometimes the news is bad, and we have beds to change over and relative value unit (RVU) targets to meet! Is there really time for compassion and empathy in healthcare? How can we be compassionate, empathetic, clinically competent, and still make budget? *Heartwiring*.

From improving clinical quality, patient outcomes, and satisfaction, we'll explore how *Heartwiring* pays dividends in performance and productivity across a wide range of clinical settings. *Heartwiring* also helps the clinical providers themselves. With compassion fatigue and burnout at record levels, we look at *Heartwiring* as a strategy to provide a valuable tonic for the chronic stress of many healthcare settings. Could *Heartwiring* return some of the joy to healthcare? Can it help with the scourge of burnout and return skilled associates to full capacity? Healthcare providers will always be under certain stress. Providing medical care will always carry a certain degree of risk. Those we care for will be stressed. But those of us who choose to work in this challenging field are up to the task. Just as technological capabilities are continually improving, we need to continually improve and evolve the human side of caring. Research shows exciting possibility in this area from a deeper understanding of the value of relationships, to evidence that empathy can be taught, to a clear picture of how the human side of healing impacts the bottom-line.

We will push for a new world order that sees healthcare as a team sport with both patient and provider on its roster. Teams caring for and with patients will become the norm in various settings including the hospital, a patient's home, and outpatient programs. Teams will be supported and connected by substantive human connections, supported by modern electronic information and communication methods, and financed by a value-based payment. Teams collaborating to provide compassionate and coordinated high-quality, appropriate, and cost-effective care across the healthcare system continuum will be required. *Heartwiring* is the solution.

Our ultimate goal is for every patient to experience the best of what healthcare has to offer from individuals as technically proficient as they are compassionate and empathetic. When a fellow human being is ill, hurt, and suffering, we should lead with compassion and empathy standing as the foundation for the clinical wisdom and technical skills needed to heal. This is what we mean by being *Heartwired*. Many healthcare administrators and clinicians have contacted us after reading *If Disney Ran Your Hospital*. They count themselves among those who have gone beyond reading and have adopted the *9½ Things* into their workplace culture. They continue working toward long-lasting and sustainable change. For them *9½ Things* was not just a period of "buzz" about the next best thing in healthcare. They are *Heartwired*.

As more and more healthcare providers become *Heartwired* the win-win-win of benefits for patients, providers, and the healthcare system will be the norm. In a *Heartwired* hospital everyone from clinicians, support staff, and administrators alike is guided by genuine compassion and empathy. As *Heartwired* clinicians, the patients we care for are not merely customers but people we know and care about. Their individual stories can be shared as often as their age, gender, major medical diagnoses, and current medications. Our ability to heal is enhanced when we forge genuine human connections along with surgical repairs, intravenous medications, or a course of physical therapy. And patients are not merely satisfied, but die-hard fans, loyal to the system and the clinicians who are *Heartwired* toward truly patient-centered care. If there is any pixie dust to be had in healthcare, our bet is on *Heartwiring*.

SECTION I

WHY HEALTHCARE NEEDS TO BE *HEARTWIRED*

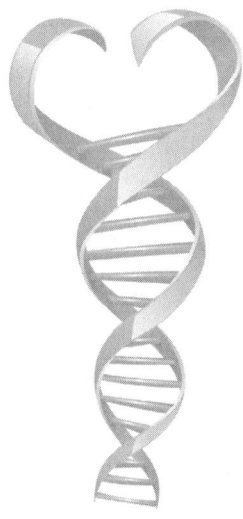

"The greatest thing in this world is not so much where we stand as in what direction we are moving."
~ Johann Wolfgang von Goethe

CHAPTER ONE

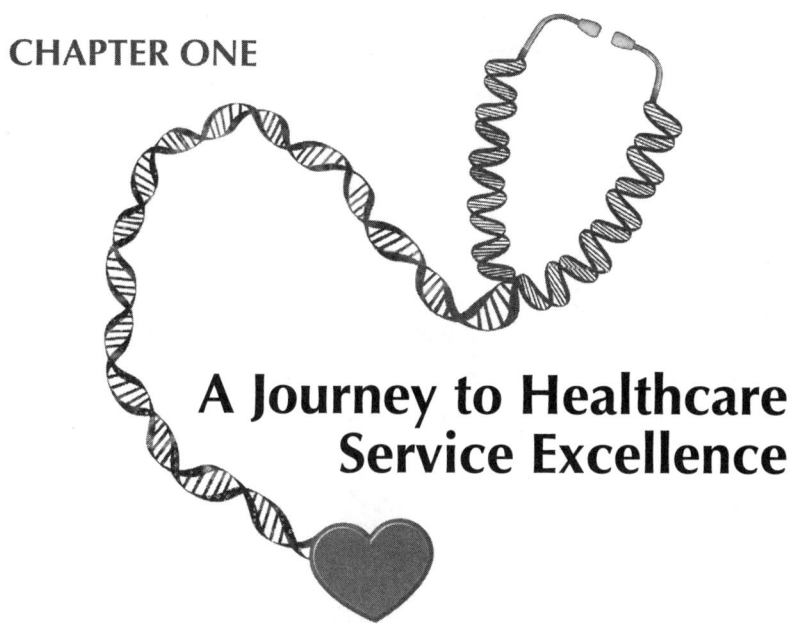

A Journey to Healthcare Service Excellence

Fred's career in healthcare spanned a transformative time in the evolving field of customer service. From the emphasis on marketing in the 1970s to the hardwired era of the 2000s, his early insights led to the *9½ Things* and his later work rounded out his convictions about the path best taken toward lasting customer service excellence in healthcare.

THE JOURNEY OF HEALTHCARE SERVICE EXCELLENCE

1966	Donabedian's Model of Quality Care
1975	Marketing & DRG's
1985	Satisfaction Surveys
1995	Service Excellence Training / Quality Improvement PDSA
2005	Patient Experience
2015	Hardwiring & HCAHPS
2020	Heartwiring
2030	

Hospital marketing was first espoused as the bedrock of connecting to customers through persuasion—how people's beliefs, attitudes, and motivations are influenced. In those days marketing was about the "Four **P**s": **P**roduct, **P**lace, **P**rice, and **P**romotion. Then came the fifth "**P**,": **P**ositioning, which was the forerunner of branding. Finally, a sixth "**P**,": **P**eople, was added, and Fred found his niche.

Early on, Fred learned the difference between marketing and selling: *"Marketing is not selling. Selling is trying to get people to want what you have. Marketing, however, is trying to have what people want. Our reputation is built more on what our customers say about us than what we say about ourselves. Their word of mouth makes selling and advertising virtually unnecessary."* That would remain his "North Star," and helped drive him toward finding more substantive ways to connect healthcare systems, including their clinical providers and other associates, to customers.

SERVICE EXCELLENCE TRAINING

With an eye toward improving the performance of associates across healthcare systems, it became clear, specific training in customer relations was in order. For the clinicians, their core competency was based on clinical skill, but patient perceptions of their care included more than that. For the Adventist Health System, an all-day employee program was created called **SHARE** and focused on developing five key skills and attitudes:

SKILL	ATTITUDE
Sense people's needs before they ask	Take Initiative
Help each other out	Teamwork
Acknowledge people's feelings	Engaged Empathy
Respect the dignity and privacy of everyone	Uncommon Courtesy
Explain what's happening	Clear Communication

Others were doing similar programs in their organizations. Attesting to the broad interest among healthcare providers, commercially available programs came on the market as well. Many of these early programs took their lead from an unlikely source, the American industrial engineer and statistician W. Edwards Deming.

QUALITY IMPROVEMENT MEETS PDSA

Though his work would influence healthcare many years later, in the 1950s W. Edwards Deming was a government statistician. He was asked by the US Government to help with the census in Japan. While there he also taught the Japanese automobile executives about process and quality management in their production plants. This guidance is credited with allowing Japan to beat US car manufacturers in quality outcomes by building quality into every process step instead of relying on quality inspectors at the end. Deming would go on to be credited with altering the course of organizational management principles across many industries and governmental agencies, including healthcare. In his final book, *The New Economics*, published in 1993 not long before his death, Deming said 85 percent of quality problems are caused by management, not workers. He put frontline employees in charge of improving quality by applying several simple analytical tools in a four-phase quality improvement process called PDSA (Plan, Do, Study, Act).

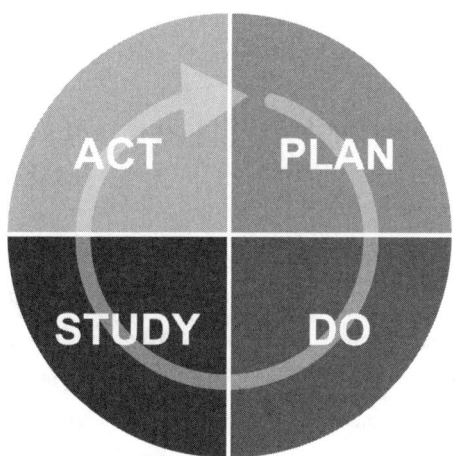

This is a simple yet powerful process of iterative change, accountability, and improvement. It wasn't long before it was the standard across many industries including healthcare.

HOW HOSPITALS MISSED THE "T" IN TOTAL QUALITY MANAGEMENT

In the 1990s, hospitals adopted, virtually en masse, W. Edwards Deming's systematic approach to quality improvement for factories. Referred to as "Total Quality Management (TQM)," the approach provided statistical tools for mapping, measuring, standardizing, tracking, and reducing variation in clinical and work processes. Healthcare, however, is not a factory. What suffices as ***total*** quality improvement in a factory, falls far short of ***total*** quality improvement in the therapeutic care of sick human beings in hospitals. Even the father of TQM recognized the deficiency. In his book, *Out of the Crisis*, Deming alludes to a critically important factor for healthcare providers that is often missed in quality improvement activities:

> "The most important figures one needs for management are unknown and unknowable… What is the value, for instance, of the multiplying effect of a happy customer and the opposite effect from an unhappy customer?"

PATIENT PERCEPTIONS—DEMING'S INVISIBLE NUMBERS

Clearly, Deming, who taught the importance of setting numerical standards for quality and reducing variation for quality improvement knew certain factors were not easily measured and manipulated. He did not fit patient perceptions into the same category as process outcomes. In fact, he goes so far as to say that what patients think of their caregivers and the care they received is something *unknowable*. Yet, he considered these "invisible numbers," as he also called them, to be the "most important numbers one needs for management." Deming further explicates the importance of subjective impressions in driving perceptions and creating promoters or fans (often called loyalty factors) which cannot be collected and quantified in the same way as objective data from survey questions. The following figure diagrams the important difference between these data categories. Quantitative data leads to clinical and financial outcome measurements that may lead to basic satisfaction, but it is the Qualitative data that generates perceptions within patients/customers that can drive satisfaction toward its highest level, today known as "promoters."

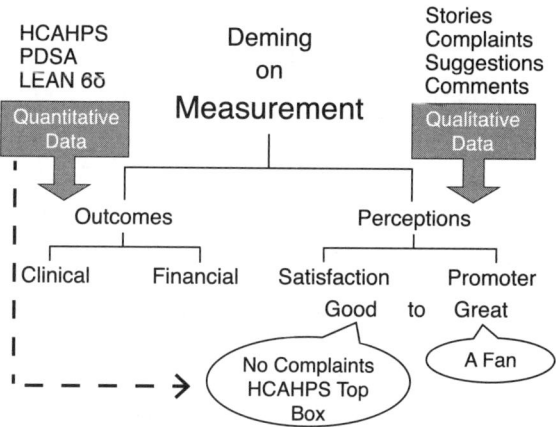

Research conducted by the Advisory Board confirmed how difficult it is to put faith in patient satisfaction scores:

1. They are subjective perceptions. Two patients can have completely different perceptions of the same interaction with staff.
2. Varying expectations mean that, aside from common courtesy, it is hard to know how much emotional support patients need or expect in any given situation.
3. Patients tend to tell us what they think we want to hear when asked, not what they really think.
4. Patients' memories fade, especially under the influence of certain pain medications.
5. Because of the complexity of care, it is hard to isolate where, when, and who a complaint or a compliment refers to.
6. Some units do not have enough responses to be statistically valid.
7. Patients hesitate to express concerns because they want to be seen as "good patients" instead of complainers.

APPLYING PSYCHOLOGY TO QUALITATIVE FEEDBACK

So how can we come to know the unknowable and understand what patients truly think about their care? How can we find the promoters? After all, we need that feedback to fuel our quality cycles. To start, we need to stop asking patients to *tell us how to improve*. Clearly, a satisfied patient has no complaints so they can't tell us how to improve. Here are two typical examples of the same question; which gets us the information we can use to improve?

> "How could our department improve our service to your department?"
>
> or
>
> "How could we have improved your hospital experience, Mr. Lee?"

On the face of it, these look like perfectly good questions. However, they both turn out to be poor questions because 90 percent of the time they will not elicit a useful answer.

The most common answer will be "I can't think of anything" because the question asks for an answer that is a "you" message instead of an "I" message. To answer truthfully means saying, "*You* could serve our department better if *you* would just_____." Or, as in the case of a patient, "You could have improved my experience if you had _____." We instinctively become defensive when we hear "You could have done X…" Any answer that starts with "You could have done X…" sounds critical and blaming. Instead of risking a confrontation with a defensive person, most of us will dodge such questions. If our questions intimidate our customers, how good is the feedback?

So, how might we frame an open-ended question so that it asks for an "I" message instead?

For internal customers (e.g., physicians): "Is there anything about working with our department that frustrates you or your staff?" The answer would now sound like this: "Well, it is frustrating when our nurses call during the lunch break and there is no one who answers the phone." Since this response asks for a frustration, it does not tell someone else how they should do their job, which avoids creating defensiveness. The asker can take the feedback to his or her department and they can decide what to do about it.

For patients, ask: "Was there anything about your stay (or visit) that frustrated or disappointed you?" With this, the responder can say something like: "It did disappoint *me* when _____." Or, "It frustrated my family when_____." Of course, we can also get the patient story by simply asking an open-ended question and giving sufficient time to listen to the answer. "Tell me all about your experience and how it felt, from beginning to end."

No doubt it is a tall order for healthcare to take responsibility for both an outcome and how an individual patient feels about their care. After all, a patient may not even care about what we know is a quality outcome, yet our responsibility includes both the outcome and their satisfaction with the care. Fortunately, strategies emerged to help manage the task.

HARDWIRING

The term *hardwiring* first became associated with healthcare performance in the late 1990s as attention to service excellence and patient satisfaction began. Baptist Hospital in Pensacola, Florida, had defied conventional wisdom by going from the percentile teens on the Press Ganey Patient Satisfaction Survey to the 99th percentile in months instead of years. Their then-CEO, Quint Studer, brought a burning-platform approach with him from his former employer, Holy Cross Hospital in Chicago, which had done much the same thing earlier. In his 2003 best-selling book, *Hardwiring Excellence*, Quint Studer introduced the concept that would revolutionize healthcare improvement efforts. When Fred first read Studer's book he thought, *finally somebody is doing in a hospital what great service companies, including Disney, have always done–require courtesy behaviors as a condition of employment!* Even the best training programs like SHARE, had made only modest improvements in patient survey results—nothing like Baptist Hospital in

Pensacola had done. The obvious difference between Baptist and everyone else, was not in what they taught in orientation and training. It was in having leaders in positions of authority that required and embodied the behaviors everyone was being taught. They hardwired their organizations and held associates accountable as a condition of employment. The rest of us were just *teaching* them and *hoping* the staff would voluntarily adopt and practice the behaviors for the rest of their working lives. Hardwiring characterizes all outstanding service organizations, whether it's The Walt Disney Company, Southwest Airlines, The Ritz-Carlton Hotel Company, or Nordstrom.

Disney cast members (all employees) had strict dress codes and were hired and held accountable by their managers for courtesy behaviors and even subjective things like *attitude*, which some employers are reluctant to address. In fact, Disney hired primarily for attitude, smiling, and natural friendliness, in the belief that it is easier to teach job competence than change personalities or attitudes. At Disney, guidelines were standards, unlike most hospitals where standards were usually treated as guidelines. For example, at the Disney Institute, when Fred was there, every cast member received a little booklet, complete with illustrations, called *The Disney Look–Appearance Guidelines*. Hospitals had something called a *Dress Code*, or *Standards of Dress*, which sounded mandatory but was treated much more like a guideline. Fred learned this subtle but clear difference the hard way.

As his tenure at Disney began, Fred was provided *The Disney Look—Appearance Guidelines* before his first day on the job. For orientation, men were to wear slacks, leather shoes, and a sports jacket with lapels. His orientation was held on a hot, muggy Florida day. Without thinking, he left his jacket in the car and strolled into "Central Casting" (Disney's Human Resources). At the registration table, the lady looked up and said, "Good morning and welcome. By the way where's your jacket?" "It's in the car in the parking lot," he replied. "I hope you can get there and back before we close the doors to the classroom at eight o'clock," she said. Fred dashed to his car and as he returned saw various attendees dejectedly leaving. There was a guy in tennis shoes, another with his zippered athletic jacket over his shoulder, and still another in blue jeans. In his first encounter with the

Disney culture, he'd learned that "guidelines" *meant* "required." *No matter what they are called*, the power of the Disney dress code to infuse a culture is dependent on consistent reinforcement by managers in every department every day.

So leaders in the healthcare industry, like Quint Studer, set about focusing on the customer by hardwiring courtesy standards, making them the cornerstone of their culture. He began by benchmarking what world-class service companies do. The first company he visited for help was Southwest Airlines. One of the things they and other great service companies were doing, where hospitals seemed weak, was realizing service and courtesy must go together—*service with a smile* from people on the phones, waiters in restaurants, clerks in stores, mechanics in a garage, cashiers at a bank, workers in a laundry. The most successful companies achieved greatness in the service industry through efficiency, timeliness, and hardwired courtesy.

For example, observe the wait staff at a fine restaurant. They *acknowledge* you with a greeting first. They *introduce* themselves. They *tell* you about the specials for the day. They give you *time* to read the menu. They keep you *informed* about delays. They ask, "Is there anything else you need?" while making it clear that they are not too rushed to serve you. They *answer* your questions about menu items and how they are made, sometimes offering to share the recipe. They do frequent *"rounding"* on their tables to see if each customer is okay. They are quick to respond if something isn't. They *thank you* for coming as you leave. By adopting the standards of the service industry and *requiring/hardwiring* them, it stood to reason that the same behaviors would make healthcare great as well.

Anyone who has worked in a hospital knows that patients want courtesy too, and until recently, we have been hit-or-miss in providing it. There was too much variation in our courtesy. We needed to be as conscientious as a waitress in meeting customers' courtesy expectations. Studer Group was formed to help hospital managers make such behaviors mandatory and hold staff accountable for them. Most hospitals recognize these behaviors, codified as **AIDET** (Acknowledge the guest by name, Introduce yourself, Duration of time involved, Explain things, Thank them for choosing our hospital or clinic). Under the banner of quality, we learned that quality is doing the right thing right, every time.

In fact, these types of *prescriptive* behaviors are universal in the service sector and customers have been conditioned to expect them, quickly becoming dissatisfied if they are not performed with a smile, even if the smile is painted on. A manager of a restaurant, for instance, requires (*hardwires*) such behaviors even when all the tables are full and there is a restless crowd waiting in the waiting area. No one is exempt from courtesy, and there is never an excuse for its absence. Now, what we expect when we go shopping or eat in a restaurant, we also expect when we walk into the door of an emergency department or a physician's office.

We expect any employee to greet us with pleasantness, introduce himself or herself, answer our questions, and return frequently to check and see if we need anything. Ringing a bell for service may have been okay for our grandparents, but we now consider it to be "poor service" if we are ignored until we ring a bell. We consider it poor service if we have to call or wave across the room in order to get the attention of a wait staff. Rounding is what we expect today—constant vigilance for signs of customer needs before they ask, even when the wait staff is rushing around with a full house.

With the growth of services, most hospitals needed a tune-up in service excellence. Nursing students and physicians, in particular, come to us straight from years of clinical training which does not typically include any training in customer service. They learned to do their technical tasks well, but since clinical competence often trumps interpersonal skills, and top leadership is focused primarily on financial performance, clinical quality, and productivity, service ended up on the bottom of their list of priorities. So, service behaviors go untaught, and clinicians end up with highly variable skills in this area.

We feel Quint Studer deserves to be in the Healthcare Hall of Fame for bringing service to the forefront and insisting that hospital managers standardize and hardwire courtesy behaviors and hold all staff accountable. In the process, he also emphasized the need to listen to, engage, honor, and thank the staff for delivering excellent service. His imprint on hospital management systems cannot be minimized and set the stage for the next level of development of healthcare service excellence.

HCAHPS: ANCHORED IN THE SERVICE PARADIGM

Anyone engaged in the work of healthcare today should know **HCAHPS** (www.hcahpsonline.org) as the government mandated patient satisfaction survey. Yet if you put the acronym in front of an audience filled with both frontline and administrative associates and ask how many can identify each word, very few outside of the quality or marketing departments are able to do it. Not even CEOs! Give it a try. How about just the first two and last two letters? HC…PS? Many guess HC stands for Health Care. Sorry, good try, but incorrect. And surely PS would be Patient Satisfaction. But that's incorrect too! HCAHPS stands for **H**ospital **C**onsumer **A**ssessment of **H**ealthcare **P**roviders and **S**ystems. While we applaud the move to encourage accountability to the end user, and many of the concepts Fred's first book promotes will lead to high HCAHPS scores, we believe many healthcare providers want to (and should want to) go beyond providing a transaction infused with simple and scripted courtesy and respect. Whether they know it or not, they are among the influencers we need in healthcare. In Chapter 5, we'll review in more depth the evidence base of psychoneuroimmunology. This field has broadened our understanding of the power of human connection. We now know deep, fully empathetic, and compassionate human interactions are a basis our healing profession requires. If we aren't careful, however, the forces promoting transactional healthcare may shift our focus too far from patient-centered, compassionate care.

In some cases, we are exchanging our venerable time-honored medical and healing lexicon in favor of the words we use in commerce and service. The root word for *patient* means "one who suffers" (from the Latin "pati"). We are changing that to *consumer*—one who purchases goods and services. The root word for doctor is *docere*, which means "one who teaches." We are changing that to *provider*—the other half of the consumer-service dyad. The root word for nurses is *nutrire*, which means "one who nurtures." Finally, as nurses are more often moved into the "provider" category as well, the shift to a service paradigm is complete. But are patients the same as consumers picking up their dry cleaning from a provider? Has the service industry given us a reason to strip healthcare of its traditional triad of:

one who suffers goes to **another** who is an authority and teacher, who relies on **another** to comfort and nurture—thus acknowledging the patient's suffering? Here a beloved physician author, Jerome Groopman, MD, expresses a similar viewpoint in *The Anatomy of Hope*:

> "What impact will this new vocabulary have on the next generation of physicians and nurses? Recasting their roles as those of providers who merely implement prefabricated practices diminishes their professionalism… We need (clinicians) with not only expertise in science and biology but also an authentic focus on humanism and caring."

HARDWIRED BUT NOT QUITE DONE YET

Improvements have indeed come from attention paid to continuous quality improvement and hardwiring excellence across our healthcare systems, but are we confident we can deliver humanistic and compassionate care like Dr. Groopman describes for each patient we encounter? A 2018 update of Gallup's annual Healthcare poll shows it's been a challenge for some time and we still have work to do. While 80 percent of Americans rate the quality of the healthcare they receive as excellent or good, these ratings "match or nearly match the averages Gallup has recorded since 2001."

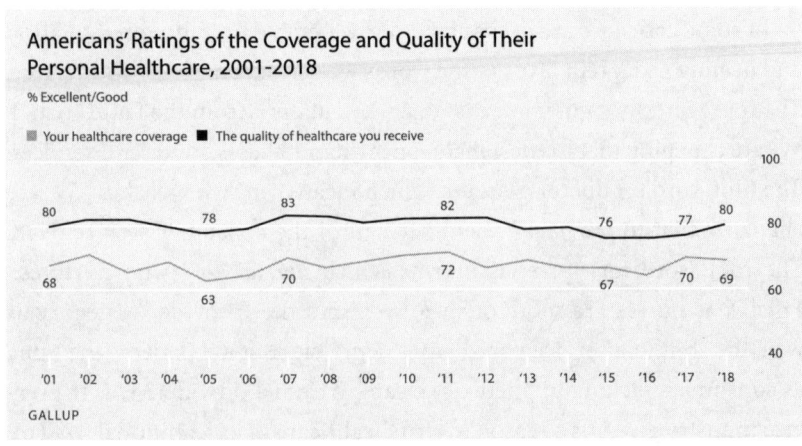

Most people who see this diagram are surprised. As we discussed earlier, many hospitals, especially the ones who have hardwired courtesy behaviors, have seen a real improvement in their HCAHPS scores. But patient satisfaction and perception of care quality is a different measure grounded on how someone *feels* about the care they have received. In the challenging arena of healthcare, it is admittedly not possible nor advisable to make everyone 100 percent satisfied. But it should be a goal to make everyone feel cared about.

We believe *Heartwiring* healthcare will lead the march to close this satisfaction gap. So how can your healthcare system become *Heartwired* and close the gap? Drop the service economy model of performance. Healthcare is more than a service. *Heartwired* healthcare organizations meet the patient, learn their story, and offer high-quality, patient-centered, compassionate and empathetic care.

CHAPTER TWO

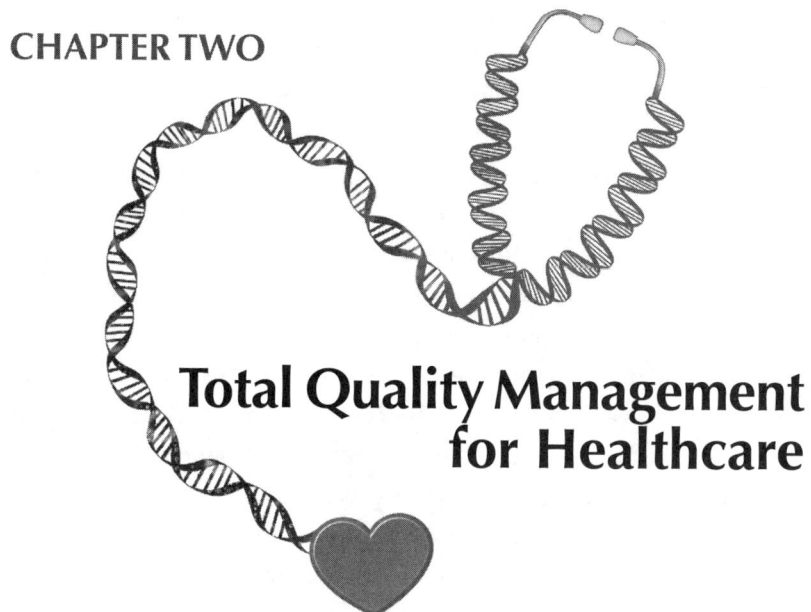

Total Quality Management for Healthcare

"Let whoever is in charge keep this simple question in her head (not, how can I always do this right thing myself, but) how can I provide for this right thing to be always done?"

~ Florence Nightingale

FRED'S EPIPHANY: "Disney World" is not a service, and neither are hospitals!

During his stint at Disney, Fred identified several critical similarities between Disney and healthcare that led him to help develop a Disney Institute program for healthcare providers. *Disney's Approach to Quality Service for the Healthcare Industry* was meant to develop a culture of accountability and performance within hospitals by infusing consistently reinforced Disney type customer service. But unlike a day at Disney, in a healthcare setting the customers aren't always happy. Walt Disney's theme park mission statement: *"We deliver fun and happiness for the whole family"* clearly does not fit the mission of a healthcare system. "The happiest place on Earth" will never describe an emergency department. Was Disney really the right model for healthcare? Fred believed it was.

Associates working for Disney and those in a healthcare system are both meeting people during a specific activity, be it going to Disney or going to the emergency department. Associate interactions present a significant opportunity to affect the perceived quality of those activities in the eye of the consumer/patient. Long-held economic thought described three active sectors—commodities, goods, and services. Disney was clearly a service. Hospitals, it was thought, were also obviously part of the service sector. And if we wanted to improve patient satisfaction, we would have to make service excellence one of our pillars of success. As Fred worked with those running the happiest place in the world, he began to understand the trip to Disney was more than a service, it was an experience like none other. And the driving force of Disney's economic engine is the *full* experience of a day at Disney, not a mere rollercoaster ride. Could the same economic engine be active in healthcare as we develop valuable, healing relationships rather than merely repair a broken wrist or eliminate elevated blood pressure?

In their groundbreaking 1999 book, *The Experience Economy*, economists B. Joseph Pine II and James H. Gilmore made a compelling case for a fourth sector of the economy radically different from the traditional three. They called it: *The Experience Economy: Where Work is Theatre & Every Business a Stage*. Throughout their book, they used Disney movies and theme parks as their quintessential example of this fourth sector.

Theater is not a Service

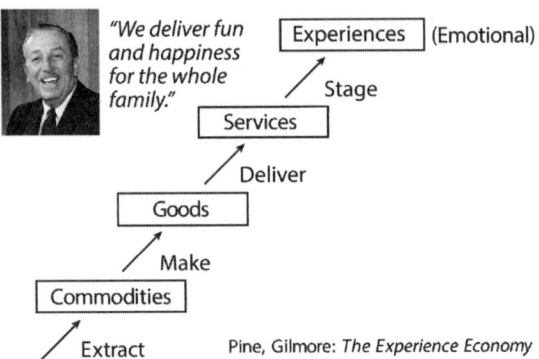

Pine, Gilmore: *The Experience Economy*

According to Pine and Gilmore, when we go to a Disney movie, park, or Broadway show, we are purchasing an experience, not merely a service. An experience is inherently emotional, and distinct from an emotionally neutral service. Nobody comes out of a theme park or a movie talking about the service they got; they talk about the *experience* they had, using words like *funny, tense, exciting, touching*, etc.

The authors defined what they meant (parentheses and italics added):

> [*The hospital, like theater...*] no longer offers goods or services alone but the resulting experience, rich with sensations created *within the customer*. All prior economic offerings (*commodities, goods, and services*) remain at arms-length, outside the buyer, while experiences are inherently personal. They actually occur *within* any individual who has been engaged on an emotional level. The result? No two people can have the same experience —period.

> ...While the *work* of the experience stager (hospital staff) perishes upon the performance [...] the *value* of the experience lingers in the memory of any individual who was engaged by the event. Most parents don't take their kids to Walt Disney World just for the event itself, but rather [...] because the value lies within them, where it remains long afterward.

In other words, commodities, goods, and services are extrinsic and temporary, but experiences are by definition *intrinsic* and leave an emotional imprint on one's memory that may last a lifetime. There's a clear difference between picking up your dry cleaning and attending a theater performance. Or dropping by Macy's to check on the current sales event and spending the day at one of the Disney theme parks. Not all experiences, like shopping, are chosen voluntarily. Not all experiences, like visiting Disney World, are happy ones. The emotional experiences of human beings (even in healthcare) can be anywhere along a continuum that runs from tragedy to comedy. Recall the symbols for *theater* are a laughing mask and a crying mask. It became clear to Fred that Disneyland®, movies, theater, *and hospitals*, are all in the same economic sector—called the "experience economy"—but meeting completely different emotional needs:

> **DISNEY:** Meeting the emotional needs of a family to have fun together.
>
> **HOSPITALS:** Meeting the emotional needs of a family going through distress, fear, pain, anxiety, and occasionally happy, but often sad, events.

Falling ill and losing one's health or mobility can be an overwhelming emotional experience. Of course, patients still appreciate any engagement that goes quickly and smoothly with friendly and helpful staff. But, unlike guests leaving a Disney movie or theme park, patients usually do not come out of a hospital raving about the service they got. They talk about the experience they had. And by experience they mean how it made them *feel*—how it met or failed to meet their *emotional* needs in a time of distress. The Pine and Gilmore model makes it clear how Disney and healthcare are similar. They both inhabit the experience economy where the emotional impact of the service provided is often the driver of customer satisfaction. *A hospital without compassion would be like Disney without fun.*

ENTER *HEARTWIRING*

Think of a physician, nurse, or therapist you know who is respected for being clinically skilled AND compassionate with patients, families, and co-workers. They are *Heartwired*! Pine and Gilmore's book introduced the experience economy where emotional aspects of the patient experience are important. For healthcare teams to move from good to great in patient perceptions, we need to develop a new understanding of this paradigm as well as the skills and attitudes to impact performance and create more *Heartwired* associates.

Look at the two pictures on the next page. One customer in a retail setting and one customer in a healthcare setting.

First, think about what is similar between them. Both customers want to be treated with dignity and respect. They both want their questions

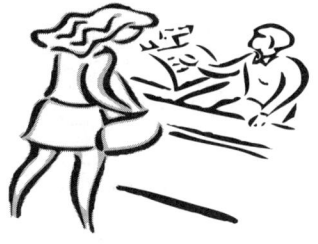 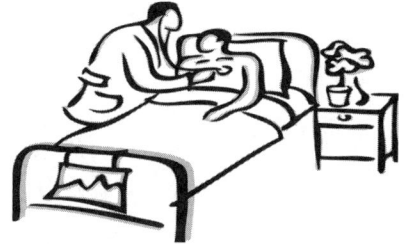

answered by a person who knows what they are talking about and can communicate clearly. They both want to know what is going to happen.

Now, think about the differences. In the first picture the customer is happy and familiar with the typical retail environment. She chooses to be there. She has done this many times before. She is dressed up, presentable, and confident. She can walk out of the store if she is not treated with courtesy. She is the one in charge. Clerks do not invade her personal space. There is no physical touching. If she wants to go to the restroom, the cashier simply points the way.

In the second picture, the healthcare customer—now called a patient—may be full of fear, worry, anxiety, and pain. He is not where he would choose to be. In fact, this is probably the last place in the world he wished to be, if he could help it. This is an unfamiliar place, and he is completely dependent. Everyone else is in charge. He is stripped of his modesty and strangers are free to touch him and probe him anywhere. If he needs a restroom, someone may have to help him *to* and *in* the restroom, or in bed by inserting a catheter, creating an uncomfortable and embarrassing intimacy.

Given the immense difference in the emotional state and needs between a person who is suffering and one who is not, it becomes clear that what makes service personnel great with their customers in a service or retail company, will not be enough to make clinicians and caregivers great in the eyes of their patients. How can we create more *Heartwired* healthcare providers?

TOTAL QUALITY VARIES BY ECONOMIC SECTOR

Every job takes a required level of competence. We hire people for their competence or we hire them because we believe they have the skills and

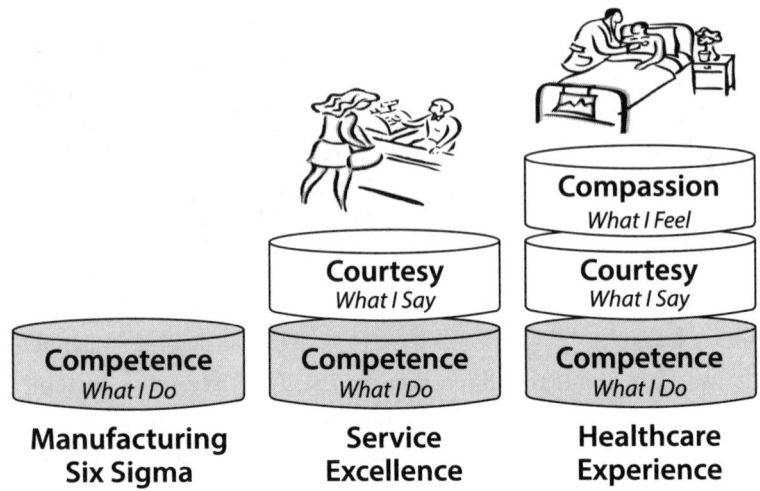

talent to develop the competence required in a particular position.

Note in the figure above, in the manufacturing sector, workers are paid *only* for their competence—the skills to do a particular task. Because they work with machines and tools, it doesn't technically matter if they are friendly or grumpy. It doesn't matter how they dress or groom. The only thing they are paid for is their competence. Quality is determined by speed, efficiency, and adherence to standards. Variations from standards and their causes are tracked and measured constantly by frontline quality improvement teams using statistical tools introduced in Japan by W. Edwards Deming called Total Quality Management (TQM) in those days, and Six Sigma today.

In the service sector, employees are paid for more than just their competence. They are dealing with a live customer, and since the customer's impression is an important condition for getting repeat business, the employer *does* care if they are friendly or irritable. Their manner and appearance become important. Dress codes, smiles, and courtesy are essential for success where customer impressions matter. Using Deming's quality improvement tools, service companies set standards of conduct, and strive to reduce variation from those standards to ensure consistency. If only some people smile and introduce themselves and others don't, there's no consistency. Without consistency in courtesy, we don't have quality service. When a customer approaches, great service organizations expect every worker to look up from whatever task they are doing, smile, and greet the customer. No exceptions. To ensure consistency, it's a great help for new service workers to be given scripts to follow.

In the experience sector, hospitals and other healthcare settings are the stage on which clinicians must deal with physical and emotional suffering and tragedy. If our goal is to facilitate "healing" rather than just "treating" the patient, it becomes essential that we engage our patients who are going through the distress of pain, fear, anxiety, and loss at the emotional level. It requires we hire people with, and/or train them to have, the skills of competence, courtesy, and compassion.

Those practicing the "healing arts" are typically focused on relieving human pain and suffering. Their tools have evolved over time from rituals performed by early Indian shamans and rudimentary surgical procedures without modern anesthesia to the intellectually and technologically sophisticated capabilities of modern medicine across the globe. In pre-modern times, physicians had become fairly good at recognizing diseases and monitoring outcomes but remained woefully ignorant about causes. As such their toolkits were lean with a limited armamentarium of medication or surgical procedures compared to modern medical standards. In the time of the Crimean War, the compassionate, observant, and ultimately iconic Florence Nightingale identified the need for a range of improvements in the care for soldiers. While she is most known as the champion of the nursing profession, an overlooked aspect of Florence Nightingale's legacy are her observations of the power of human emotion on outcomes: *"Apprehension, uncertainty, waiting, expectation, fear of surprise, do a patient more harm..."* Indeed, one can say she foreshadowed the current era in which we are uncovering the magnitude of the brain's healing abilities and the impact potential of the human connection between patient and healer.

It is said Florence Nightingale was present at the bedside to comfort nearly two thousand dying soldiers. Called the "Lady with the Lamp" she was known to walk among the soldiers at night by lamplight ensuring each knew that they were deeply cared about by those caring for them. Was she aware of the healing power of her visits? Did she know by comforting a scared soldier and bringing him calm she may have improved his chance for survival? Probably not, but her prescient leadership continues to benefit us all. Modern research has identified emotional stress to be a significant culprit to healing, actively suppressing a number of the body's repair mechanisms. While we no longer use oil lamps, we can emulate Nightingale's dedication to the patient. It would not be a stretch to say that what Florence Nightingale brought to the evolving field of healthcare delivery was far more valuable in the 1840s than anything most physicians did alone.

We now know clinician empathy improves the psychosocial context for healing. So along with training in the sophisticated medications and procedures available, we can also improve patient experience and outcomes by developing teams of like-minded, quality striving healthcare professionals who deliver care with compassion and empathy. Learning from the service sector has been a momentous step on the journey of quality improvement in hospitals, but a *hardwired* culture of service excellence, should not be the ultimate destination. Building on that paradigm, we believe creating a *Heartwired* culture and team able to readily and consistently provide quality care with compassion and empathy should be the goal. A *Heartwired* culture will lead to improved patient and family experience through teams of talented clinical and support staff practicing the full range of healing arts.

The *Heartwired* Hypothesis for Healthcare Excellence:

We have reached the ceiling in how much we can improve patient care by **hard**wiring universal service expectations.

We now need to become a culture of carers **Heartwired** to connect with our patients as individuals and provide high-quality, satisfying, compassionate, and empathetic care.

CHAPTER THREE

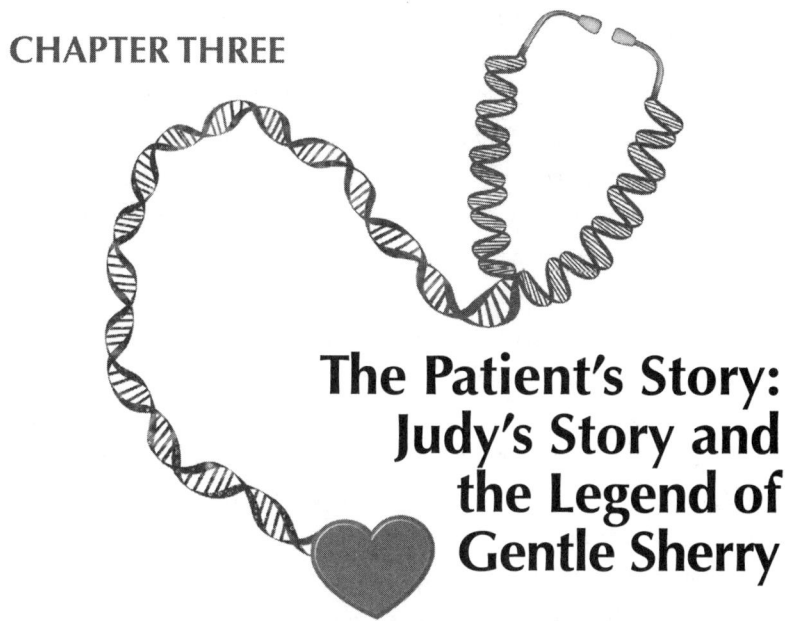

The Patient's Story: Judy's Story and the Legend of Gentle Sherry

"Tell me a fact and I'll learn.
Tell me a truth and I'll believe.
But tell me a story and it will live in my heart forever."
~ North American Indian proverb

Stories are powerful vehicles for communicating about our shared human experience. In healthcare while the specific symptoms of an illness may vary, by virtue of our shared human psyche all patients have considerable shared experience of dependency, indignity, fear, and uncertainty. As healthcare providers we must know and respect that experience. We must know and respect its impact on and implications for patients. This multifaceted knowledge, when authentic and applied, is what creates the foundation for compassion and empathy in healthcare. Here are the stories of Judy, a patient, and Sherry, a phlebotomist. Their stories teach important lessons about the role of compassion and empathy in healthcare.

Judy's Story—as told to Fred:

About five years ago I went through a very traumatic experience. I had a radical mastectomy for advanced breast cancer. The physician told me I had about three years to live. So, as you can see, thank God, I have already beaten those odds. On the day I was admitted, there evidently was no room ready for me. I waited in the hallway for hours, extremely distressed. I kept thinking about my new baby granddaughter—how she would never know me. I would just be a photograph in her mother's scrapbook. I was on the verge of tears, trying to be brave around my husband who was as devastated as I was.

Finally, the anesthesiologist arrived. "I have been looking all over for you," he said. "How come they haven't put you in a room yet?" "I don't know," I said. "I think they have forgotten all about me. I got here about three hours ago." "Well I'm going to check on that," he said, and went off down the hall. When he came back, he had a nurse with him who said, "We have a place for you, Judy." Then she took me upstairs to a little room that looked like it used to be a storage room. No windows. A bed, but no room for a chair where my husband could sit. I burst into tears. "What are you crying about?" the nurse asked. All I could say was, "Look at this room!" She said, "This is not going to be your permanent room. It will just get you by tonight until your surgery tomorrow. Then we will have a regular room for you." The worst night of my life came the next night after surgery. Even though I was in a proper room, I felt so discouraged and sad, overwhelmed with grief. I didn't think I could handle what was ahead—chemo and radiation and all the misery that goes with it. If all I had was three years and I couldn't be part of my granddaughter's life, what good was all the effort and pain? All I wanted to do was cry. But my husband was sitting beside the bed and I knew if I started crying, he would never leave, and worry over me all night. So I said, "Go home, honey, and get your sleep. I don't think I can sleep with you sitting here. I'll be too worried about you. If we are going to deal with this one day at a time, we will need our sleep. He finally got up, kissed my cheek, turned off the light on the wall at the head of the bed and asked one final time, "Are you sure?" He had no more than left when I started to cry. While I was sobbing quietly to myself, a nurse came in. She had a little tray in her hand. When she turned on the light and looked down and saw that I was crying, she turned the light off and put her tray down. She took the same chair my husband had been sitting in and pulled it right over to the bed. Then she sat down and reached for my hand. I was just trying to pull myself together for the nurse, but when she did that, I clutched her hand and wept harder than I have ever wept in my life. Even though she didn't say a word, it was like somebody finally said, *Go ahead and cry. Who wouldn't? You don't have to be brave for me.* She sat there for quite a while. I remember thinking, she can't sit here all night and hold my hand. So I pulled myself together and said, "You are an angel. You'll never know how much I needed that. Thank you." Only then did the nurse stand up, pick up the little tray, and say what I'm sure she planned to say when she came into my room, "Judy, I've brought you something to help you sleep."

As he listened to Judy, Fred was touched, "What a beautiful story, can I tell it to other people?" "Yes", Judy replied, "If there are nurses in the room, please tell them that sometimes they can be of more comfort to a complete stranger than their own families can be. I'm concerned nurses think that patients' family members are the best ones to comfort them. But what if you are worried about your family trying to cope and don't want your family to know how discouraged you are? I never thought I would ever feel that way, but the worst thing my nurse could have done is to run down the hall and bring my husband back because I was crying." "You know, Fred," she said, "You'll sleep better at night if you know your nurse really cares about you and what you're going through." "That's interesting, considering there was a sleeping pill in your story," Fred replied. "Are you telling me that what the nurse did helped you sleep more than what the physician ordered?" "Yes," she answered. "If a nurse holds your hand while you cry, you know she really cares. And when you believe your nurse really cares about you and what you're going through, you can't imagine that she could ever pass your room in the night without checking on you. That's why you can sleep. You trust her to watch over you because you know she cares about you."

"So, Judy," Fred said, "I imagine you will always have a very positive feelings about that hospital—maybe for the rest of your life." She shook her head, "No, I can't say that I have positive feelings about that hospital, even though I loved that particular nurse, and I will never forget her." "Really? I often say that one person's actions can give a halo effect to the whole organization."

"I'm sure that's true if *all* your experiences are good. But I think other people can cancel it out. Remember that first nurse—the one who put me in a storeroom on my first night? Well, she turned out to be the nurse manager on my floor. I will never forget what she said to me when I left. My husband was pushing my wheelchair, and everybody was saying goodbye to me. Then the last thing I heard was that nurse calling after me, "I will never forget you, Judy. You are the only patient I ever had who cried about a room!" "I was mortified," Judy continued, "I probably won't ever forget that remark or the nurse who said it. I wasn't crying over a room. I was crying because my wonderful life was being ripped apart by cancer. It was like my tears were behind a dam, ready to burst at any moment. The room was just the last straw in a horrible day, and all those tears that had been in check for weeks, suddenly came pouring out."

THE *HEARTWIRING* CONNECTION

When Fred told Judy's story to his wife, Aura said that the nurse who had dropped everything to connect with Judy emotionally actually did something clinically important and impactful. "During the unit on psychoneuroimmunology (PNI), we learned how stress affects the immune system. I tell my nurses that because compassion and empathy reduce a patient's distress, it is *part of their clinical practice*, not just part of being courteous.

Courtesy alone has no clinical effect, but really connecting with the patient at an emotional level often does. So, the fact that this nurse took the time for compassion, means she was doing something often better than any medication a physician can order."

That is why compassion, not necessarily clinical skill, was the first thing Aura looked for when she interviewed a new nurse applicant. She knew that starting with a smart and compassionate new nurse, deliberative training paired with appropriate mentoring and modeling would develop a high-quality and compassionate nurse every time. She knew that basic knowledge and skills are relatively easy to develop, but attitudes, kindness, and compassion aren't as easily developed by repetition alone. If compassion is missing, patients will know it, and no protocol you put in place will disguise it. As Aura experienced, "There is no way you can set a standard for every way an employee might make a bad impression." Scripts can tell a person what is required to say, but scripts do not typically come with guidance for tone of voice or other non-verbal messaging. During interactions with patients and families, it is often something non-verbal like facial expression, body language, or tone of voice that imparts the emotion of the moment. Patients may sense your compassion, understanding, and acceptance through what you say and how you say it. But just as easily, patients can sense condescension, disapproval, and displeasure. In fact, when words conflict with affect, either visually or in tone, we have all learned to believe what we see or feel over what we hear. As we are becoming *Heartwired*, we will learn about how to best communicate our compassion and empathy. For now, understand the powerful connection between our thoughts and behaviors.

All emotions and behaviors come from our thoughts or imaginations and the feelings they trigger. So, ultimately, it is what we think and imagine that governs body language. We may intend to be nice and kind, but if we imagine that the patient is an annoying crybaby, it will color our non-verbal cues, even when we try not to show it. Lie detector devices rely on the fact that most people cannot successfully pretend something they do not feel. It's like blushing. All the effort in the world to not blush cannot overcome the feelings that make you blush. We have little conscious control of our non-verbal cues. People always seem to always know when we are faking it. Judy certainly did.

On our path toward becoming *Heartwired*, the good news here is that knowing this connection, we can take advantage of it for good. Have you ever seen one of those smiley face stickers placed near a phone? That's to remind everyone to smile while speaking, allowing positive emotions to travel across the phone line. Try it, it works!

The Legend of Gentle Sherry

In 2011 Fred was invited to give a talk at a TedXMaastricht in Maastricht, Netherlands. The following is an excerpt from that talk. To see the full TedX, see:

https://innovativehealthcarespeakers.com/speaker/fred-lee/

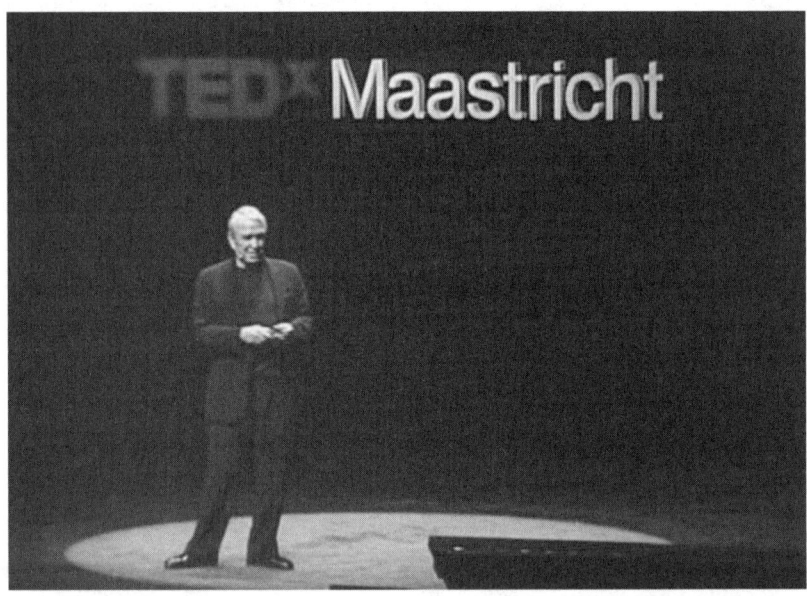

Let's pretend I am lying in my room, having just been admitted to the hospital. A pleasant person walks in, smiles, and says her courtesy script, "Good afternoon, Mr. Lee. My name is Sherry. I'm from the lab and I am here to get a blood sample from you."

I say, slightly concerned, "Good afternoon, Sherry. They already drew my blood when I was in the emergency room. Do you really have to do it again? Doesn't it all go to the same lab?"

She sets her tray down and says, "I don't know about that. I just know I'm supposed to get a blood sample from you. Maybe they need to check on something that was not ordered with the first sample. Besides this will only take about five minutes and I have been doing this for many years, so there's nothing to worry about."

THE escalating tension in a period of SILENCE

I extend my arm. She is now silent, intent on her task. We are both silent looking at the crook in my arm where a needle will soon be inserted.

What happens during silence just before an invasive procedure? Our minds will go where every patient's mind goes just before *any* invasive procedure. I wonder if this is going to hurt. It shouldn't, but sometimes things can go wrong. My mother told me when I was about nine years old that they could put a bubble in your arm which can go straight to your heart and kill you! This person could *kill* me!

What else could go wrong? Did you know they could blow out your vein? How does that phrase sound–**blow out your vein**? Do you know what they say when they blow out your vein? I heard it once, "Ooops!" How does that sound during an invasive procedure? Then the person looks up and says, "I think I blew out your vein!" As you wince and blink, she adds, "Give me your other arm!" If I have ever had someone miss my vein, it gets anchored in memory, and will taint my perceptions every time I get my blood drawn. Will they find my vein on the first stick? If they miss the vein, how many more times will they try? And how many times will I say, "Ouch?"

If these are the thoughts going through my mind, which are the natural kinds of thoughts in anticipation of any invasive procedure, what is happening to my blood pressure? To my pulse? When the blood pressure and heart rate go up, what happens to my pain threshold? It goes down, which means that everything feels like it hurts more because even a small amount of anxiety reduces a person's tolerance for pain. Everything hurts more when we are not relaxed.

She puts a rubber strap around my bicep. Something really hurts! I look down and see that she has caught some of my skin in the knot. I'm sure she will release it and start over. But instead, she just tightens it down. OUCH! What goes through the patient's mind at this point? I can tell you. *"If she can't see my skin in the knot, how will she ever find my vein?"* I look at her face and it has a frown on it. What does a frown tell you when the person is looking for something? When she reaches for the syringe, I don't think she has found the vein. All my senses are focused on the certain likelihood that she will surely miss the vein on the first try. I steel myself for the inevitable. At this point most people would look away, not wanting to actually watch the phlebotomist miss their vein. They would be tense; time suspended. BANG! The needle strikes. It feels so big. I glance and see that she found the vein! Eureka! On the first stick no less. *How lucky was that?* All the while she's thinking, *How great was that? First stick. The patient must be impressed.*

She wraps up, "Is there anything else I can do for you?" She has said her script, checking off the courtesy box. And she got the sample on the first stick, which means she was clinically perfect. Can't get better than that. Or can it?

Let's pretend someone is making rounds with a clipboard and enters my room just as the phlebotomist leaves and says, "Hi, Mr. Lee. I'm Susan, the team leader tonight and I want to be sure we are *always* treating you *excellently*. Was that the lady from the lab? Did you just have your blood drawn?"

"Yes."
"May I ask you a few questions about her performance?"
"Sure. Go ahead."
"Did she smile and was she friendly when she came into the room?"
"Yes."
"Did she use your name and introduce herself?"
"Yes, she did."
"Did she tell you why she was here and what she was going to do?"
"Of course."
"Did she answer all your questions in a way you could understand?"
"Yes."

"Did she get the vein on the first stick?"
"She sure did."
"So, would you say she was excellent?"
"By all means. She was perfect."
"Can you think of anything she could have done to improve your experience, Mr. Lee?"
"Absolutely not. As I said, she was perfect." (And I would mean it.)

Sample survey done. Top box. Satisfied patient. Perfect!

Still, does being perfect in every way you can measure automatically create a loyal customer or fan?

The answer is really quite simple. Here's the test: If I am satisfied and don't care who comes back tomorrow, I am not particularly a fan of Sherry.

Let's replay the experience and notice some subtle, but important differences.

Same courtesy script (which is always essential). Sherry enters, greets me by name, introduces herself, explains why she is here and what she is going to do, and answers my question about using the draw they took upon admission.

But instead of professional silence:

Sherry observes my state of mind and notices that I am a bit tense. So she distracts me by asking something like, "Do you live around here, Mr. Lee? Or do you come in from out of state like a lot of patients do this time of year?"

No, I live around here. Been here many years. Raised two kids who live here too."

"What do they do?"

"My son works for Apple. My daughter, who went to college as pre-med with math and science scholarships graduated Summa Cum Laude, and is now a very fine artist!"

"Wow." She puts the rubber band on while I proudly add, "Even Tom Hanks owns one of her paintings." She knots the strap. I don't notice the pinch because I am trying to make a point. Did she hear Tom Hanks?

Sidebar: Notice that Sherry invites me to fill the silence instead of filling it herself. She could have gone on and on about her own life. But if she does the talking, it doesn't distract my mind. It is easy for me to fake listening, especially if underneath it all I am in a nervous state of mind. I can go right on nodding and smiling without hearing a word.

Sherry might add some more calming reassurance for the heart rate and blood pressure. "You've got a good vein here, Mr. Lee. I should have no problem with this one."

I say, "Are you sure? I don't see a vein there."

She says, "We don't look for veins, we feel for them. It's right here. Wanna feel?"

"No! I don't want you to lose it."

She decides on bit more reassurance, "I've been doing this for fifteen years," she says. "Beginners can be a little rough. But in the lab, I am known as Gentle Sherry."

I smile. "I got Gentle Sherry?" (what did that just do to my heart rate and blood pressure?)

She puts the needle on top of the vein. I don't feel a thing yet, but I see blood seeping into the vile. "Wow, how did you do that?" I ask.

"Told you," she says.

She wraps up with her script. "Before I go, Mr. Lee, is there anything else I can do for you?"

"Well, I can't think of anything right now, Sherry," I say, "But if somebody has to do this again tomorrow will you please be the one? Don't send Rough Rudy up here. Or some beginner!"

Gentle Sherry was *Heartwired*. The nurse who held Judy's hand was *Heartwired*.

They understood the clinical *and* emotional needs of their patient, and completed their clinical task with appropriate efficiency and compassion. We are sure you know some *Heartwired* associates in your healthcare system. Seek them out. Engage them in a training and mentoring program. You've no doubt heard that smiling is contagious, right? So is *Heartwiring*. These associates can help you spread *Heartwiring* across your system until it's the defining characteristic of your culture of compassion and empathy. It's time to take what we know about what our patients need and put into practice processes that allow us to close the gaps between what we know and what we do.

CHAPTER FOUR

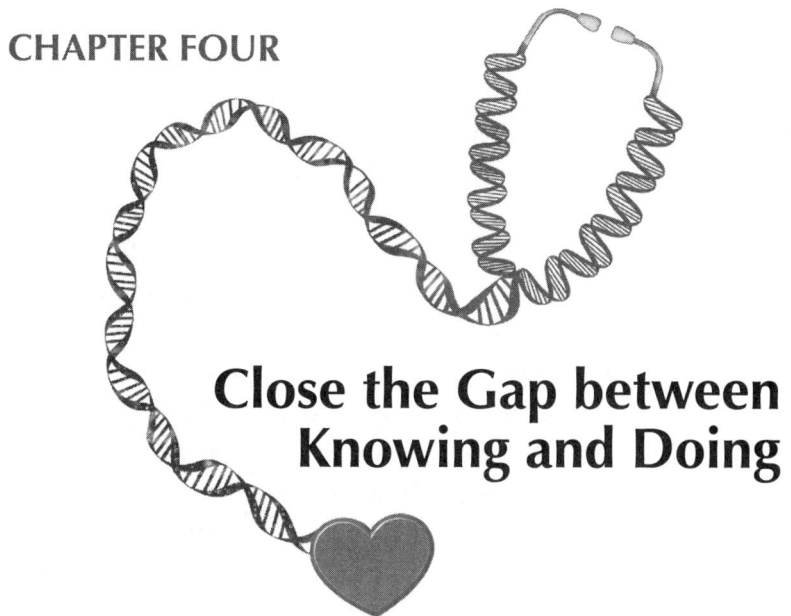

Close the Gap between Knowing and Doing

"Don't just talk the talk...walk the walk"
~ author unknown

Here's the playbook we've all been looking for. Lest we remain in a perpetual cycle of one-off customer service "sure bets," we need to close the gap between what we know our patients want and need, and what we do to meet (or exceed) those expectations. As we journey toward being *Heartwired* for excellence, let's see what it takes to close this crucial gap.

Does Disney have the secret sauce? What separates Disney from all the other wannabes in the experience economy is not Disney's unique knowledge about what customers want. It is Disney's consistency in the day-to-day management of universally shared values and commonly desired behaviors. Like Pete Sampras and Serena Williams, two of the greatest tennis players of all time, Disney does all the same things everyone else in their field does, but Disney does them more consistently, especially under pressure, and over a longer period of time. That's the secret sauce. These are the qualities that separate champions from the rest of the pack.

This gap between knowing and doing—or knowing and performing with high quality and consistency—is not easy to close. Especially in an organization lacking a culture aimed at excellence with processes for continuous quality improvement and managerial accountability. Sometimes we pin our hopes that a different consultant will have the secret. Sometimes we try over and over to close the knowing-doing gap without changing the deeper things that cause the gap and keep it stubbornly in place. They are like a talented tennis player constantly looking for the coach that will have the secret to winning without hard, grueling work. Maybe there is a special shot. Maybe there is a secret strategy. Maybe there is a miracle diet. But more than likely, it is thoughtful, hard work that is required for success.

The gap between knowing and doing is not easy to close, but there are strategies that can help. First, you must create an infrastructure supporting performance excellence. To describe why the infrastructure is so important, let's use a common example of enforcing a dress code. Once you have your infrastructure, we will describe the four major strategies you can use to close the gap and start walking the walk.

Figure 4.1: Performance Model (Part 1)

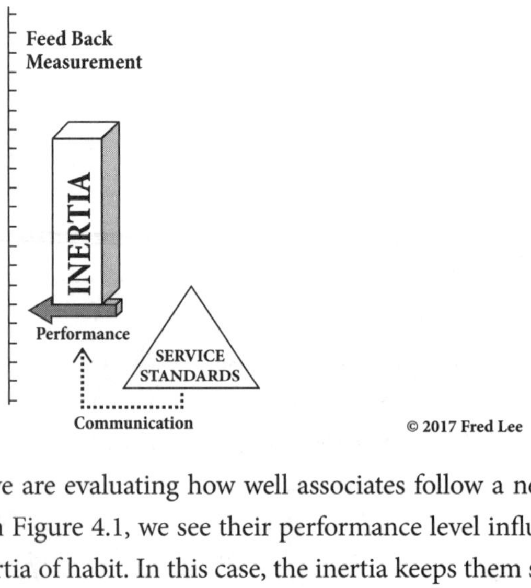

© 2017 Fred Lee

Imagine we are evaluating how well associates follow a newly required dress code. In Figure 4.1, we see their performance level influenced by the weight of inertia of habit. In this case, the inertia keeps them stuck wearing their old uniform, not the new dress code. Next, imagine they are sent an email reminding them of the new dress code standards. For a period of time and among some associates improvement is observed (see Fig. 4.2). But how likely is that method to inspire widespread and sustained performance improvement? Most of us would answer that neither is likely. We might then try a training program during a mandated town hall or team meeting. If these training programs have outstanding trainers and the content receives high marks from the attendees, there is often a bump in the scores. Good, that seemed to do the trick. Feedback data begins to show an upward trend, and optimistic administrators hope the trend will continue. The trouble is, it *never* does. As dress code violations increase, committees are set up to figure out what is happening and how to keep employees compliant. In our model, committees are part of the triangle labeled "service standards." Committees churn out dress code standards. Does that do the trick?

Look at the model again and notice that the connection between service standards and associates is shown as a *dotted* line. At best a great program has some influence (dotted line), but *absolutely zero solid-line authority over those who attend.* That's right: zero-line authority. With no authority over employee behavior, how can the inertia of poor habits ever be overcome? With no authority, trainers and committees are left only with cajoling as their main technique to affect change. Let's add the missing element to our model: Leadership, see Figure 4.2. Only directors and managers have authority over performance and can affect change.

Figure 4.2: Performance Model (Part 2)

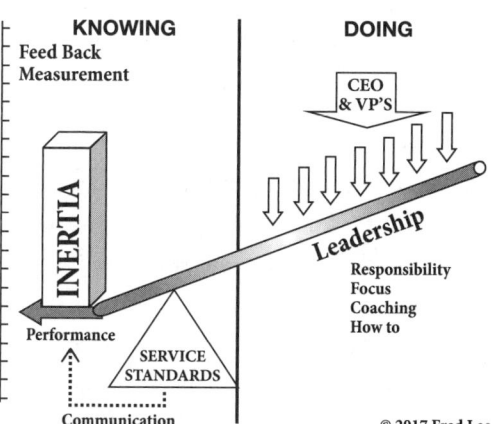

With leadership added to the model, let's now review four strategies that support change efforts.

Strategy 1: Leadership Accountability

"Accountability breeds response-ability"
~ Steven Covey

This model puts the major elements of performance improvement in the right relationship. It does not show that programs are not important or should be abolished. It doesn't diminish the role of inspired committees or motivated employees. It simply shows that reading vision statements, knowing patient expectations, hearing stimulating stories, and learning communication and attitude skills are the *fulcrum*, not the *lever* for improvement. Whenever efforts are made to improve patient experience there are common questions that come up over and over: "Are our managers going to pay any attention to this?" "Will we have enough resources to really make the change?" And finally, all too often, "Are the physicians going to go along with this program?" Leaders promoting change need to be knowledgeable, invested, engaged, and supportive of the associates who will actually make the changes matter to the ultimate outcome of excellent patient care.

Strategy 2: Systems Do What Systems Measure

"There is no secret to success. It is the result of preparation, hard work, and learning from failure."
~ Colin Powell

As a health system vice president once said so bluntly and correctly, "My people do what I tell them to do. If I pay attention to something, they will too. Otherwise they won't." That is the stark reality in a nutshell. Outcomes that show up on the dashboard and are reviewed by the whole team, get the time and attention of management. Choose items carefully and strategically. Plan rapid and repeated PDSA cycles across a range of settings. Install term-limits for key indicators that need quick improvement. Manage the improvement and then move on to other areas of need.

Strategy 3: Avoid Paralysis by Analysis

"When all is said and done, more will be said than done."
~ Aesop

How much information or knowledge is needed to find ways to improve healthcare delivery for patients? Collecting feedback does not in itself cause actions to be taken on the feedback. Most hospitals have a process to obtain patient-satisfaction feedback, yet how many actively take action that eliminates the problem or improves the system? It is a trap to believe that knowledge is a force for change or action. Action comes about by *doing*, not by knowing or thinking or planning or listening or talking. In fact, the most effective ways of doing are learned from trial and error, not necessarily from knowing *how* before one starts to *do*. PDSA cycles from Deming's TQM are a good example of this iterative process.

As Jeffrey Pfeffer and Robert I. Sutton write in their book, *The Knowing-Doing Gap: How Smart Companies Turn Knowledge into Action:* "One of the most important insights from our research is that knowledge that is actually implemented is much more likely to be acquired from learning by doing than from learning by reading, listening, or even thinking. Spend less time just contemplating and talking about organizational problems. Taking action will generate experience from which you can learn."[1]

Strategy 4: Use Failure for Good

*"Failure is simply the opportunity to begin again,
this time more intelligently."*
~ Henry Ford

A potential barrier to taking action is the possibility that the experience will be a negative one. Thomas Edison famously said of his invention of the light bulb: "I have not failed. I've just found 10,000 ways that won't work." "Many of life's failures are people who did not realize how close they were to success when they gave up." Within healthcare the allowance for failure has limits of course, but the lessons of failure analysis shouldn't be ignored. We need to thoughtfully and honestly examine our "failures" if we ever hope to improve systemic deficiencies in patient care, patient experience, and health system operations. In her article in Harvard Business Review, April 2011 edition, Amy C. Edmunson describes the challenge and opportunities well: "My research has shown that failure analysis is often limited and ineffective—even in complex organizations like hospitals, where human lives are at stake."[2]

"Few hospitals systematically analyze medical errors or process flaws in order to capture failure's lessons." Research in North Carolina hospitals, published in November 2010 in the New England Journal of Medicine[3], found that despite a dozen years of heightened awareness that medical errors result in thousands of deaths each year, hospitals have not become safer. Fortunately, there are shining exceptions to this pattern, which continue to provide hope that organizational learning is possible.

At Intermountain Healthcare, a system of hospitals that serves Utah and Idaho, physicians' deviations from medical protocols are routinely analyzed for opportunities to improve the protocols. Allowing deviations and sharing the data on whether they actually produce a better outcome encourages physicians to buy into this program.[4]

In Figure 4.2 (page 39), pay close attention to the line separating those activities that are about *knowing* and those that are about *doing*. Avoid the temptation to focus on the "knowing" side and do all you can to move to the "doing" side. Take action! Leaders need to set the pace and lead all associates to take responsibility for walking the walk, focusing on what's most important in the customer's experience, coaching others, and doing the things that win the hearts of customers and staff. With this type of leadership, you will close the gap.

CASE STUDY: How Holy Cross Hospital Closed the Gap

Holy Cross Hospital in Chicago was the first large, urban hospital to receive national exposure for going from the lowest quartile in patient satisfaction to the very top among the approximately four hundred hospitals in the Press Ganey database at that time. For them it was the simple fact of survival for the board, the CEO, and the entire management team. Being at the bottom can do that. It can create a real crisis not felt in hospitals that are already pretty good compared to their competition.

Liz Jazwiec, then director of the emergency department at Holy Cross, has remained an active change agent for improved patient experience.

Everyone wants to hear her tell about going from being the worst emergency department in patient satisfaction to one of the best. She readily admits that she was a skeptic at first. When her boss said, "There's no reason that you can't be as good as Disney World at customer service," she thought he was completely out of touch with reality. "You want to see Disney World?" she would say, "I'll show you Disney World. Come down to my department some Friday night about one A.M. We've got Adventureland. We've got Never Never Land. We've got Tomorrow Land. We've got Fantasy Land. We've got the whole thing for you."

When the rest of the hospital went from the 14th percentile in patient satisfaction to the 75th percentile in six months, the emergency department was still at only the 8th percentile. Liz took that as validation that their department was the only department doing the real work of saving lives and stamping out disease. Obviously, everyone else had time for that service fluff, but her people didn't. Her boss was not pleased. He gave her two choices, either believe in the goals and follow the program, or leave. "Unless you drastically change these scores in ninety days, you're fired," he said. In the meantime, he moved her replacement into her office. Without a choice, she did it, pulling off what she considered to be impossible. Whenever anyone asks Liz Jazwiec how she caught the vision of service excellence and where she learned the leadership skills to make such spectacular improvement in only a couple of months, she admits that she did not read any books or go to any seminars. "I was nearly fired, twice," she tells them candidly.

One word succinctly summarizes a key difference between hospitals that receive high satisfaction scores and those that don't: *hardwired*. When responsibility for satisfaction is hardwired into every manager's accountabilities, then courtesy gets hardwired into every employee's performance evaluation. As Liz says, "We do what we are held accountable for doing." Hardwiring is an essential element of efficiency and quality. It can take a poor culture and make it better, even good. And hardwiring then sets the stage for moving to what we believe is the next level of service excellence, *Heartwiring*.

In the next section, we set our sights on how healthcare leaders and associates can each inspire and lead their teams to move from being hardwired for service excellence to being *Heartwired* by contributing to the development and growth of a culture intent on delivering high-quality, satisfying, and compassionate care.

SECTION II

HOW TO *HEARTWIRE* HEALTHCARE

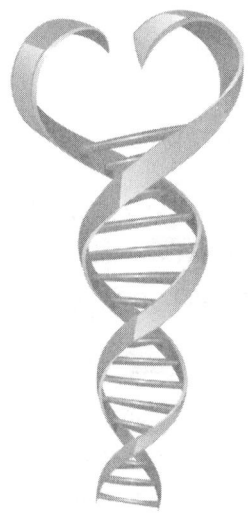

*"I've learned that people will forget what you said,
people will forget what you did,
but people will never forget how you made them feel."*
~ Maya Angelou

In Section 2, we move from theory to action. How can we become *Heartwired* and lead others in that direction as well? First, we explore the basics of human interaction and the origins of a model of interpersonal interaction now well known as the bio-psycho-social model. Groundbreaking in its day, it began the push of clinicians toward more personal rather than solely technical encounters. We will review recent evidence of just how active the mind-body connection is in regulating physical and emotional states. For modern-day healthcare workers who want to perform at their highest level, and clinicians who wish to heal with compassion and promote whole-person health, learning to be *Heartwired* is the key.

As social beings, human interactions have a broad and direct influence over our general well-being and health. *Heartwired* associates will need to carry new skill sets that include the knowledge, skills, and attitudes of promoting healthy mind-body connections. The ability to create a positive therapeutic connection between a healthcare provider and patient can mean the difference between health and disease. Think that's touchy-feely nonsense or want to pass it off as unsubstantiated hogwash? Read on for an updated perspective on mind over matter and a new understanding of placebo.

No longer regarded as underhanded trickery, we have a far more sophisticated understanding of placebo and its potential for altering a physical process. Well beyond its use as a sham pill, researchers have identified that the provider-patient relationship itself is part of the "placebo effect" and through that connection, a unit of change. Beyond the pill or surgery, the relationship takes an active role in therapeutic outcomes. A *Heartwired* provider can be just the therapeutic ally a patient needs. Nurses or therapists can communicate and interact with patients in specific ways to make success more likely. Did you know a smile contains a certain amount of the cure? A patient's positive attitude can reduce stress and allow the immune system to function more effectively. As patients do the work of healing, we can help them by being *Heartwired*.

Next, we will explore the process of *Heartwiring* healthcare associates with a foundation of compassion and empathy to guide and enhance their performance. Is compassion innate or can it be a learned skill? What about empathy? Are some of us born to care more than others? To begin, we define these uniquely valuable but commonly confused attributes and evaluate their role in the patient experience. Then we look at strategies to promote the development of healthcare providers as skilled in compassion and empathy as they are in the specific clinical aspects of their roles.

To further develop clinicians with empathy, we will look to the emerging field of narrative medicine that is illuminating the value contained within key aspects of our patient's story and how such a story influences a patient's experience. Often forgotten in the sterility of medicine is the context of illness within a human story, a human life. Who is this person with pneumonia? Is it a "hot gallbladder" in 430A? No! It is a married 44-year-old university professor and mother of two with her second bout of acute cholecystitis (an acutely painful infection of the gallbladder). What does the patient want? How does this illness affect her, her family? What is she hoping for, fearing, expecting? Along the way we will meet several patients and hear from administrators working to improve their care. In most cases, throughout the book, we've changed the names to protect privacy, but you will also see we've included the names of patients and healthcare administrators who wanted their story to further this vital message. Knowing and appreciating our patient's story is indeed a necessary tenet of being *Heartwired* and propels us toward more effective points of interaction with our patients.

CHAPTER FIVE

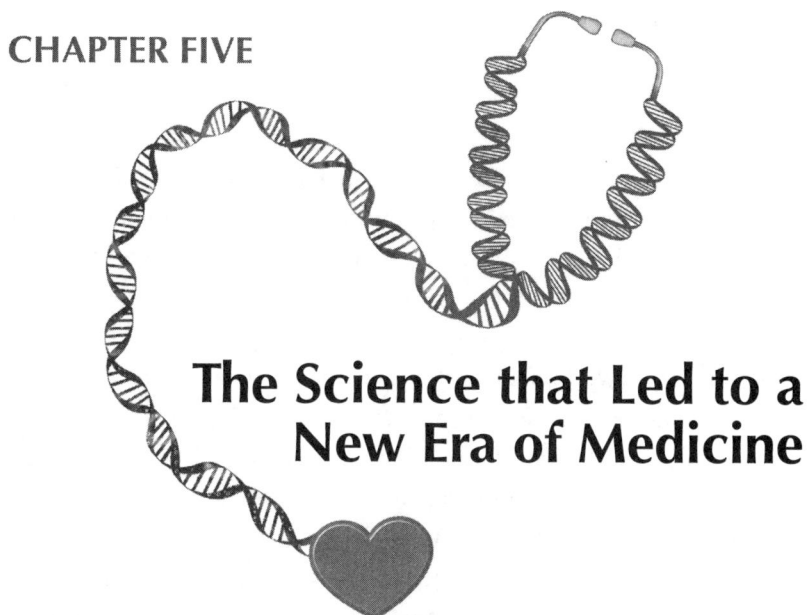

The Science that Led to a New Era of Medicine

"Most people never pay much attention to the ultimate source of a happy life, which is inside, not outside. Even the source of physical health is inside, not outside."
~ 2016, Dalai Lama speaking to Archbishop Desmond Tutu and Douglas Abrams in The Book of Joy

The Yin and Yang of the Stress Response

Believe it or not, we owe our current understanding of the mind-body connection to an unlikely source, namely stressed-out rats. In the 1930s Dr. Hans Selye, a newly minted endocrinologist and assistant professor at the University of Montreal, began a series of experiments using rats to learn more about the role of sex hormones in humans. With limited funds for his nascent research efforts, he followed a tip from a tech in a neighboring lab and acquired an extract from rat ovaries that no one knew anything about. Afterward, he set about injecting rats with the extract every day to see what would happen. Amazingly, the injected rats developed peptic ulcers, had greatly enlarged adrenal glands, and shrunken immune tissues. He had seemingly discovered the effects of the mysterious ovarian extract. Being a good scientist, however, he'd run a control group: rats injected daily with saline alone, instead of the experimental extract. At the study's end, the control rats had the same peptic ulcers, enlarged adrenal glands, and atrophy of tissues of the immune system. Dr. Selye reasoned through these results. The physiological changes couldn't be due to the ovarian extract after all, since the same changes occurred in both the control and the experimental groups. Was there something else the two groups of rats had in common?

As he pondered this question, one aspect of the protocol stood out. Every day, Dr. Selye and his assistants manhandled, dropped, chased with a broom, cornered, pinched, upended, and generally terrified all the rats in both groups in order to stick them with a needle. The poor creatures began to panic when even his shadow entered the room—little hearts pounding, little lungs gasping for air, little eyes wide open with fear and anxiety. The ulcers and altered immune tissues appeared to have been triggered by something other than the experimental extract. He next postulated that it was emotions like discomfort, fear, and anxiety that were the real culprit here. To test this theory, he put some rats on the roof of the research building in the winter, others down in the boiler room. Still others were exposed to forced exercise, or surgical procedures. None was given an injection. In all cases, he found increased incidences of peptic ulcers, adrenal enlargement, and atrophy of immune tissues.[5]

We now know exactly what Dr. Selye was observing. He had discovered the biologic cascade of stress-related hormones. It's now clear his discovery was the tip of the iceberg. Stress hormones are a complex network that are both life-saving and critical for acutely maintaining organ system equilibrium, but almost inexplicably also capable of creating long-term damage when expressed chronically. Conditions impacted negatively by stress include cardiovascular disease, obesity, peptic ulcers, and depression. Stress is also known as a trigger leading to process dysfunction at a cellular level, for example, contributing to poor wound healing and lowered immune response. As we have come to a more sophisticated and complete understanding of the role of stress in our physiology it is all the more critical that healthcare providers become more adept as agents promoting healthy stress balance. *Heartwiring* is a calming step in the right direction.

STRESS HELPS AND HARMS

While admittedly an oversimplification, your mind and body's adaptive response to stress can have both positive and protective effects along with damaging and, in the extreme, fatal effects.

In its earliest description, the "fight or flight" reaction was described by Harvard professor Dr. William Bradford Cannon in the early 1900s.[6] He identified the immediate survival benefits that a stress reaction can trigger. Hormones are released making our heart rate increase. The increased pumping action leads to delivery of a greater supply of nutrients to muscles allowing the needed burst of speed to flee danger. Clearly this is a protective and desired response. Through the earlier work of Dr. Selye, however, we also came to understand the physiology of a response to stress that is sustained chronically. Remember Dr. Selye's rats were stressed out daily for weeks. Under those conditions he found enlargement of the adrenal gland, atrophy of the thymus, spleen, and other lymphoid tissue, and gastric ulcerations. Dr. Selye called it the General Adaptation Syndrome, and though there were later refinements of his initial theories, it gave the first glimpse into the potential negative effects of stress response.[7]

If the stress response is turned on repeatedly, or if you cannot turn off the stress response at the end of a stressful event, the stress response that can save your life can also do real damage to tissues and organ systems. A large percentage of what we think of when we talk about stress-related diseases are disorders of excessive stress responses. To better distinguish the good and bad stress, Dr. Selye coined the word "eustress" for positive responses to stress. There is a eustress sweet spot where our stress response has maximum benefit as shown in the following figure. Your response to stress in running, sports, public speaking, and weightlifting, for instance, can make you better, stronger, and faster by promoting increased attention, more rational thinking, and emotional balance. Unfortunately, too much stress moves into the "distress" category where your attention is spotty and excess excitement or burnout contributes to disorganized thinking and behaviors.[8]

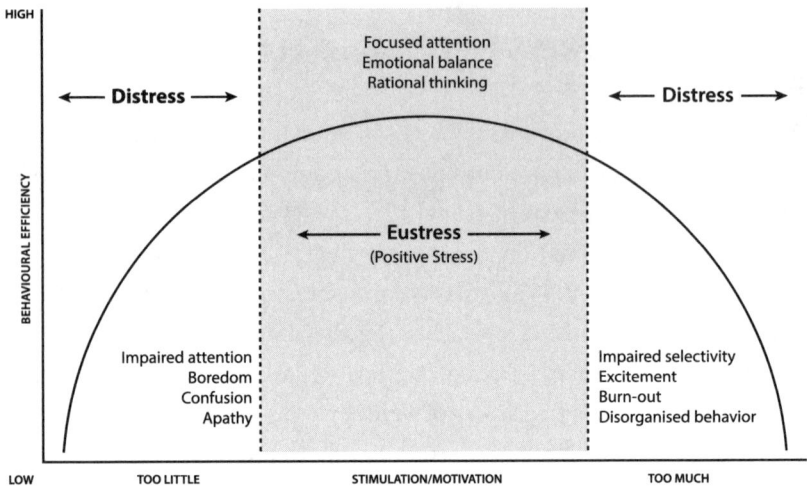

For an in-depth, graduate level book on all the mechanisms, pathways, immunological, and pharmacological agents the body uses to deal with distress and disease, we highly recommend the exceptionally fascinating book by Robert M. Sapolsky, *Why Zebras Don't Get Ulcers: The Acclaimed Guide to Stress, Stress-Related Diseases, and Coping*. While doing some early research for this book, Fred had the privilege of attending one of Dr. Sapolsky's seminars as he explained the title and themes of his book:

> To start, I must call forth a concept from ninth-grade biology—homeostasis.
>
> A stressor is anything in the outside world that knocks you out of homeostatic balance, and the stress-response is what your body does to reestablish homeostasis. But when we consider ourselves and our human propensity to worry ourselves sick, we have to expand on the notion of stressors merely being things that knock you out of homeostatic balance. A stressor can also be the anticipation of that happening. Sometimes we are smart enough

to see things coming and, based only on anticipation, can turn on a stress response as robust as if the event had actually occurred. Some aspects of anticipatory stress are not unique to humans—whether you are a human surrounded by a bunch of thugs in a deserted subway station or a zebra face to face with a lion.

Psychological stress is a recent invention, mostly limited to humans and other social primates. We can experience wildly strong emotions shockingly similar to those of a savanna baboon who has just lunged and slashed the face of a competitor. And if someone spends months on end twisting his innards in anxiety, anger, and tension over some emotional problem, this might very well lead to illness.

Dr. Sapolsky's main lesson is this: if you are a zebra running for your life, or a lion sprinting for your meal, your body's physiological response mechanisms are superbly adapted for dealing with such short-term physical emergencies. For the vast majority of beasts on this planet, stress is about a short-term crisis, after which it's either over with or you're over with. When we sit around and worry about stressful things, we turn on the same physiological responses—but they are potentially a disaster when provoked chronically. A large body of evidence suggests that stress-related disease emerges, predominantly, out of the fact that we so often activate a physiological system that has evolved for responding to acute physical emergencies, but we turn it on for months on end.[9] Building on the work of Drs. Selye and Sapolsky, let's next explore in more detail the impact our mind can have on two specific systems of the body critical to emotional and physical well-being.

In 1975, after demonstrating classical conditioning of immune function, psychologist Robert Ader and immunologist Nicholas Cohen of the University of Rochester coined the term Psychoneuroimmunology (PNI) to describe the study of the interaction between psychological processes and the nervous and immune systems of the human body.[10] The main interests of PNI are the interactions between the nervous and immune systems and the relationships between mental processes and health. Ader and Cohen, along with neuroscientist Dr. David Felten, went on to edit the groundbreaking book *Psychoneuroimmunology*, which laid out the underlying premise that the brain and immune system represent a single, integrated system of defense.[11] Evidence supporting their thesis has emerged.

Marucha and Kiecolt-Glaser reported in the *Journal of Psychosomatic Medicine:* "Dental students took an average of 40 percent longer to heal a small, standardized wound made prior to examinations, compared with an identical wound made during vacation, and their production of interleukin-1, an integral for the healing process, was reduced by two-thirds."[12]

When facing upcoming exams, stress hormones modulated their immune systems in such a way as to deplete certain cell types needed for wound healing. With a limited supply of the cells needed for tissue repair, it took longer to heal the wound. After completing exams and heading off for vacation stress hormone levels declined, the immune system returned to usual function, and wounds were healed.

Since this early description we have come to understand that the connection between an individual's mental processes and healing can be affected by thoughts they have themselves, but apropos to our work promoting *Heartwired* healthcare, the connection can also be affected by interactions *between* human beings. We call this psycho-**social** neuroimmunology.

THE PSYCHO-SOCIAL-NEUROIMMUNOLOGY OF *HEARTWIRING*

Our heart beats approximately 115,200 times a day, and is the body's key physiologic workhorse. We've also given it symbolic stature symbolizing our emotional core. As we've learned, strong internal connections exist between how our body functions and our brain thinks and feels. Our intellect and emotions impact physical function in both distinctly measurable (e.g., heart rate) and more subjective ways (e.g., rate how you feel on a scale from one to five). In our development of healthcare workers and teams that are *Heartwired*, the *heart* is our shared humanity and the *wiring* refers to both our personal psychoneurological connections and those *bonds* we can choose to forge between ourselves and our patients. Let's explore how this new understanding can help us evolve our delivery systems from hardwired and quality based to *Heartwired* healthcare associates engaging with empowered patients in a collaborative effort to improve their health and well-being.

HARDWIRING is *solo*—and focused on the providers needs or the needs of the system.
- I will say _____ to achieve the desired outcome I am seeking.
- I will act in the most efficient and cost-effective manner.

HEARTWIRING is *dyadic*—and focused on the patient and the provider's needs.
- I will listen for _____; I will say _____ to know and understand this patient in order to achieve good outcomes for this patient and myself.
- I will adjust my actions to care for this patient with compassion and quality.

HARDWIRING is checklists, scripts, surveys, tasks, and procedures people are required to follow.

HEARTWIRING is professionals within a culture of compassion displaying authentic empathy and engaging with patients in their care.

Heartwired healthcare professionals listen, relate, assure, and care because they believe that to be their role and duty; and they see "success" as both a well-cared-for patient *AND* a well-performed act of healthcare. In an article entitled *Ten Principles for More Conservative, Care-Full Diagnosis*, Gordon D. Schiff, MD, et al. reference the benefit to health systems that "maximize relational and informational continuity" noting they "perform better and cost less."[13] How we inspire and lead more members of our organization to be *Heartwired* should be the number one activity of leadership.

CHAPTER SIX

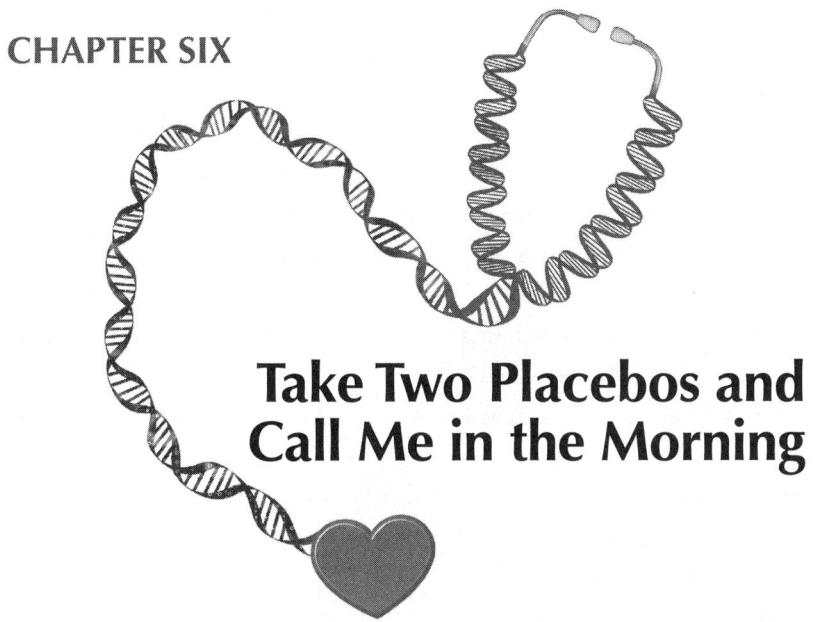

Take Two Placebos and Call Me in the Morning

"Cure sometimes, treat often, comfort always."
~ Hippocrates

In his outstanding lecture series called *Mind-Body Medicine: The New Science of Optimal Health*, Jason M. Satterfield, PhD, faculty member of the University of California, San Francisco School of Medicine, uses the foundational science of the bio-psycho-social model[14] to explain the interconnectedness between those factors about us ("bio" and "psycho") and our world ("social") that contribute to our personal journey of sickness and health. Learners come to understand "how the 'outside' (e.g. stress, relationships, work) gets 'inside' to alter the functioning of our minds and bodies." In hospitals and other healthcare settings this knowledge is emerging as a critical component of the skill set for anyone coming into contact with patients and their caregivers. Indeed, as we will learn a *Heartwired* healthcare provider with compassion and empathy within their skill set is more likely to be effective in modern healthcare delivery.

Let's look in more detail at why this would be. How would a *Heartwired* physician result in patients with more self-confidence and self-worth who also end up better able to control their diabetes? Why do the patients of *Heartwired* nurses calm more easily and sleep better in the noisy environment of a hospital? What is it about being *Heartwired* that makes an individual physician or nurse or administrator so powerful? Increasingly, research is uncovering evidence that the human interactions making up the "patient experience" are actually part of a critical and active component of the "therapeutic relationship" that can profoundly affect our patients' outcomes for better or worse. It's crystal clear. It's the relationship and interactions between two human beings that is the foundation of how we think, feel, and ultimately behave.

How involved are our thoughts in creating moods and behaviors? Some seem obvious. If I am thinking of a pet I've lost, I feel sad and I might feel my eyes tear up. When frightened, a universal behavior is to shield the eyes. So if thoughts can create emotion and trigger behavior, can they also direct how we *feel* about a situation such as a medical therapy? And more overtly, can these *feelings* impact the outcome of a medical therapy? The answer to both questions is yes.

An experience from Fred's youth gives a clear example of the power of the mind to impact emotions and ultimately to impact the perceived effectiveness of a medical therapy.

As Fred recalled the story:

> "When I was a boy in the 1950s I was bitten by a dog with rabies. We were living in Taiwan at the time because my parents were American missionaries. While playing in the streets I saw some neighborhood kids throwing stones at a shivering dog cornered at the intersection of two walls. I couldn't bear to hear the dog yelping in pain, so I rushed in to save the poor creature, and carried it home. Over the next few days my mother helped me feed and care for the dog, but it responded by snarling and snapping at us. After we had been bitten several times, we became concerned. It didn't take long to discover that the dog had rabies. Soon after that, our Chinese physician told us we would have to have a series of rabies shots–one a day for two weeks. The shots seemed huge to me and were very painful. Even though my mother set a stoic example, I cried out in pain. She agreed that it hurt and comforted

me. The next day, I begged the physician to let my mother give me the shot. Thankfully, the physician knew my mother was a nurse and agreed. I will never forget what a difference it made when it was my mother–instead of the physician–giving me my shot. It just didn't hurt near as much. I could easily "take my medicine like a man," when she gave me the rest of my shots, moving carefully from place to place so as not to hit a tender spot from previous shots."

What Fred had experienced was something medical science now knows as a ***placebo effect***. Not merely a "sham pill" used in clinical research trials, the placebo ***effect*** is a multi-faceted dynamic interaction between clinician and patient that can impact the therapeutic outcome. This may in fact be where *Heartwired* healthcare can have its greatest effect. Brain scans and hundreds of recent scientific studies have expanded our understanding of the psychosocial dimensions of pain, illness, and healing. What happened to Fred was not imaginary. There was a measurable physiological response to his mother's kindness and commiseration. Recent research reported by Gallup researchers in their bestselling management leadership book, *First Break All the Rules*, shows this effect is not limited to mothers and sons.

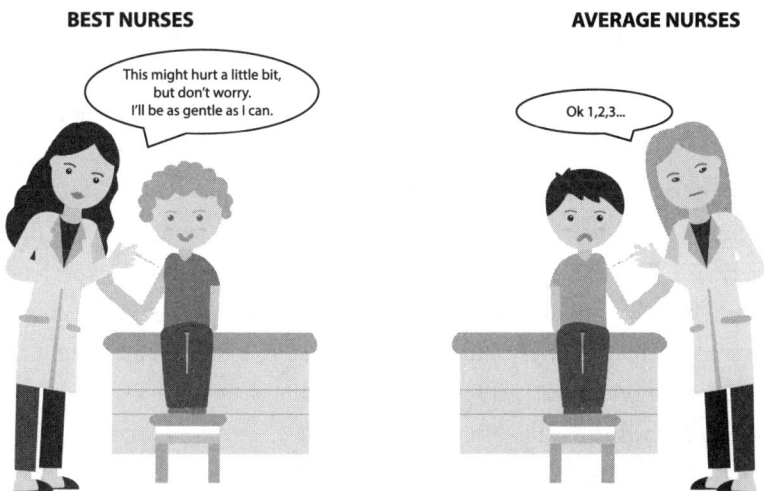

Two groups of nurses were chosen to give identical placebo shots to patients. One group was identified as "best nurses" based on patient compliments. The other group identified as "average nurses" was made up of nurses without any record of either compliments or complaints. Both groups of nurses injected the same one hundred patients in a double blind, randomized order. After each nurse left, the facilitator asked the patient to rate the pain of the injection. Although the procedure was performed in the same way, with the same dose of the same saline solution, the "best nurses" received much lower pain ratings than "average nurses."

Viewing videos afterwards, researchers concluded that the only explanation for this discrepancy was in what the nurse said just before inserting the needle. Unlike their counterparts, the best nurses said something designed to reassure and calm any fear the patient might be feeling, like, "This might hurt a little bit, but don't worry. I'll be as gentle as I can." The researchers concluded that: "The best nurses were blessed with the relating talent of empathy… To the patients it seemed as though the nurse was, in some small way, going through the experience with them. The nurse was on their side. The nurse understood. So, when the needle broke the skin, somehow it didn't feel as bad as they thought it would."[15]

The impression that the nurse "was on their side" may have had less to do with the actual words she used, than with her tone of voice, eye contact, facial expression, and body language. We use verbal and non-verbal cues to infer another person's emotional state or intentions. Research has shown that a patient exhibiting anxiety or fear will quickly calm when they perceive their caregiver has genuine concern for them. This calming effect has been shown to lower the heart rate, blood pressure, and pain threshold. Fred's mother and the best nurses knew to use empathetic words and actions to help their patients avoid a stress state that would worsen their experience. They still got a shot which surely hurt a bit, but the experience of that shot was not as painful. It is clear the ability to help patients feel better and achieve better outcomes works before a painful procedure. As we explore provider-patient relationships further let's also look outside the realm of procedures. These days, while advances in robotic surgery grab a lot of headlines, the healthcare more people in the world need comes from a seemingly simpler source, a conversation between two people.

Let's think about high blood pressure, for example. It is one of the leading chronic conditions in the world. For most patients, there is no surgical cure for their high blood pressure. A mix of changes in personal lifestyle and medication are the key interventions leading to successful control. Does the provider-patient relationship matter for these interventions? Absolutely! Remember earlier when empathetic nurses were able to make a shot less painful for their patient? Interactions between healthcare providers and patients can result in a change in the patient's physical state. Just how powerful is the interaction? Could it be that the interaction itself between healthcare provider and patient is a unit of healing? Evidence is mounting that the answer is, "yes."

In their groundbreaking article, "Placebo Effects in Medicine," Drs. Kaptchuk and Miller broaden the concept of placebo beyond its depiction as a sham pill. The "placebo effect" is "an improvement in the patient's symptoms attributable to their participation in the therapeutic encounter with its rituals, symbols, and interactions.[16] In the April 2012 *Harvard Health Letter* article, "Putting the Placebo to Work," Dr. Kaptchuk explains the current understanding that some of the "placebo effect" is "a favorable reaction to care and attention from people who patients believe can help ease their suffering and distress. An effect of care that's caring." He goes on to detail a study that illustrates the point and provides evidence of the effect. Researchers associated with Harvard's placebo studies program published a study in 2008 involving Irritable Bowel Syndrome (IBS). Volunteers for the study had IBS, a condition that causes abdominal pain and changes in bowel movements in the absence of any discernible changes to the bowel. The placebo treatment was sham acupuncture, using needles that, unbeknownst to the patient, retract into their handles instead of penetrating the skin. An impressive 44 percent of those treated with the sham procedure reported relief. The placebo effect at work. Even more impressive however, when sham acupuncture was combined with attentive, empathetic interaction with the acupuncturist, the placebo effect got even larger with 62 percent reporting relief.[17] Research is starting to show that these placebo effects are associated with detectable changes in brain chemistry that explain, in some part, the subjective improvements. This bears repeating. Placebo effects create detectable changes in brain chemistry that explain why people feel better. A placebo effect is a REAL improvement in how a patient feels. Yes, it may be "all in their head," but they aren't faking it. They *are* better! Research in pain treatment and depression has shown the natural pain–relievers, called endorphins, are released in response to placebos. So our caring and creating positive therapeutic encounters is not just icing on the cake to ensure five stars on HCAHPS, it is an active part of the healing process for our patients. Creating a positive therapeutic encounter should be considered step one as we interact with patients.

THE POWER OF THE PLACEBO EFFECT

As we've learned from Drs. Kaptchuk and Miller, the placebo effect is real and when a provider-patient relationship is attended to carefully it can leave patients having "a favorable reaction to care and attention from people who patients believe can help ease their suffering and distress. An effect of care that's caring." Caring can, in fact, be the first step on the road to recovery.

SILENTLY SUFFERING

Consider Mrs. "G", a pleasant and friendly 69-year-old woman. She and her 43-year-old disabled daughter, Amy, recently moved to Florida. They moved to be closer to her eldest daughter, Jennifer, who is an RN. One day they all came to a specialty geriatric clinic for an evaluation of recent problems Mrs. G was experiencing with her memory. Mrs. G's medical history included major depression, diabetes, and obesity. Recently, Jennifer could tell her mother was suffering great stress as the main caregiver to her sister, Amy, who herself was developing multiple medical issues further complicating her disabilities. Approximately one year ago, Mrs. G lost her husband of 48 years, and since, has seemed even more stressed. Most concerning were the memory lapses and unexpected cognitive difficulties Jennifer had observed in her mother over the past year as the move was being arranged.

In the first clinical visit Mrs. G, a former university librarian, was a lovely and pleasantly sociable woman who admitted to recent forgetfulness and finding it surprisingly difficult to learn her way around her new neighborhood. She was not taking her medications regularly and admitted she "always carries around a lot of stress everywhere I go." Her past history included a bout of depression successfully managed with counseling and medication. As the evaluation progressed, it became clear that her mood was an active issue. The diagnosis of major depression was reached after she reported several weeks of low mood, changes in sleep, loss of pleasure in her usual hobby of needlepoint and a completely uncharacteristic lack of desire to leave her new home or meet anyone new. She was referred to a counseling service and prescribed a previously effective antidepressant.

Mrs. G returned in six weeks with Jennifer. She had begun the medication but had chosen not to start counseling. She reported feeling much better. Her daughter estimated there was a "90 percent improvement." When Mrs. G was asked what she thought had helped her so much, she told the physician, "It was you and coming here." She went on to explain that her former primary care provider in Wisconsin, was "very good and nice enough, but I never felt I could really talk to her or that if I did, she'd never think of me the same way afterwards." "I hadn't told her how much I miss Dan or how worried I'd become with all the trouble with the move. And I didn't want her to think I couldn't handle caring for Amy. But here, everyone seems like they really care about me, no matter what."

What is going on here? What contributed to the 90 percent improvement? Most people hearing this story give full credit for the improvement to the pill. There is evidence to support improvement from medication, though, a 90 percent improvement is much better than the research shows likely.[18] But perhaps her improvement was all due to the medication chosen and had little to do with the patient/physician interaction. Stopping at this interpretation misses a critical lesson about the value of being able to create an effective interpersonal relationship with patients. The presence of an effective working relationship between a provider and a patient is the necessary foundation for positive therapeutic encounter.

How did it come to pass that the PCP in Wisconsin (Physician 1) was unaware of the symptoms of major depression? Did she miss the diagnosis? No, she was never told the symptoms! Mrs. G was suffering in silence; she didn't feel comfortable enough to divulge her symptoms. And because she did not report her symptoms there was no chance for Physician 1 to help her achieve relief. What about the medication that Physician 2 prescribed?

Maybe that is where all the 90 percent improvement came from. Even if we assume that all of the reported improvement came from the pill, the prescribing of the pill only happened because the patient felt comfortable enough with Physician 2 to reveal her symptoms. It was the overall positive "therapeutic encounter" that led to a successful outcome. This type of "therapeutic encounter" is a new part of a broader definition of the "placebo effect." A growing body of research has identified that our ability to create a positive therapeutic encounter plays a significant role in our ultimate abilities as healers.

In the *New England Journal of Medicine* article, "Placebo Effects in Medicine," Dr. Kapchuk summarizes the role of the placebo effect in creating active therapeutic alliances between patient and provider:

> Placebo effects are often considered unworthy and illegitimate. They are thought to be unscientific and caused by bias and prejudice. This attitude obscures a core truth of medicine: medicine's goal is to heal, which can include cure, control of disease, and symptom relief or provision of comfort. When no cure is available —an inevitable occurrence at some point—medicine's ultimate mission is to relieve unnecessary suffering. Supportive and attentive healthcare (preferably with effective medications, but even without) legitimately creates a "therapeutic bias" in patients toward hope and an experience of relief and reprieve. Research suggests that distinct neurobiologic mechanisms are activated. Empathic healthcare creates a cognitive–affective–sensory orientation, tapping into conscious and nonconscious mechanisms that can predispose patients toward reduced symptom severity and lessened reactivity to underlying pathophysiology. Or to borrow terms from the behavioral social sciences, healing interactions "frame," "anchor," or "nudge" patients toward shifts in their perceptions of their symptoms and illness, making them less disturbed or perturbed. This shift is part of medicine's moral imperative to relieve unnecessary suffering in a manner consistent with trust and transparency.

Achieving this type of actively therapeutic relationship will be a challenge for all of us practicing in the high-demand, value-based world of healthcare today. After all, you have to be—at the same time—compassionate, empathetic, up to date, and evidence based but open to patient's input, technically proficient, time sensitive, and culturally sensitive, appropriate, and open-minded. What? Is this possible? Yes, highly compassionate physicians like this exist. Patients know who they are. And it makes a difference for their care. The physicians identified as displaying high levels of compassion have better care outcomes than physicians identified as low compassion. Patients of highly compassionate physicians were more likely to have optimal blood sugar control and lower odds of serious complications.[19][20]

These high compassion providers are *Heartwired*. They have been able to provide high-value and evidence-based healthcare while at the same time exuding compassion for their patients. We believe *Heartwiring* healthcare will ultimately help move our modern and advanced healthcare system forward. It will be a powerful combination if we can bring a culture of *Heartwiring* forward alongside the tremendous scientific and clinical excellence that US healthcare is known for. And how does one create a culture of *Heartwired* healthcare providers? Though challenging to achieve, the recipe is clear: **Compassion + Empathy = *Heartwired*.**

In the next chapter as we discuss compassion and empathy in detail, we will learn from the leading authority on empathy, psychiatrist Dr. Helen Riess. A turning point in her career came during a study in which her encounters with patients were videotaped. As she studied the interactions between herself and a particularly challenging patient, she saw something she had not detected during the clinical encounter. It was evident from the biometric monitors (e.g. heart rate) that the patient was experiencing significant anxiety. Dr. Riess, a trained and experienced psychiatrist, had missed it. Talk about suffering in silence! That is when Dr. Riess began the work now known as Empathetics to help those of us in healthcare recognize the emotional cues that can lead us toward deeper, more accurate, and more effective therapeutic relationships. Unless we can create alliances that are authentic and rooted in our patient's reality of their life and sickness, we will be less effective than we'd like to be.

CHAPTER SEVEN

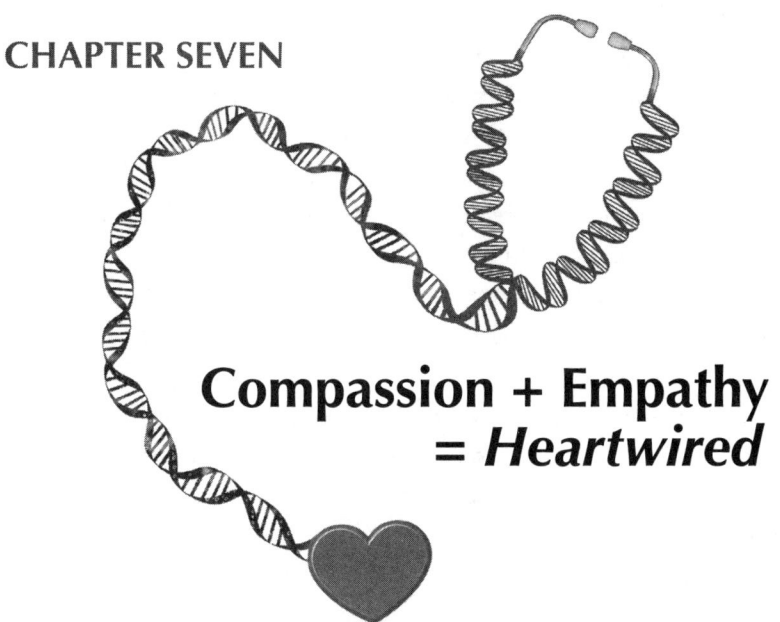

Compassion + Empathy = *Heartwired*

*"If you could stand in someone else's shoes…
Hear what they hear. See what they see. Feel what they feel.
Would you treat them differently?"*
~ Cleveland Clinic, 2013 https://www.youtube.com/watch?v=cDDWvj_q-o8

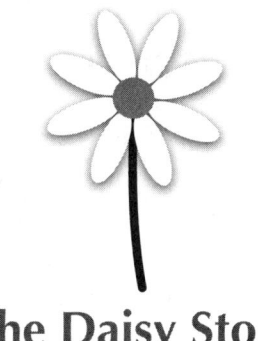

The Daisy Story

During her tenure as Director of Nursing, Aura, Fred's wife, asked a nurse to offer an opening meditation at a staff meeting. When called to begin, the nurse came forward and stood in front of the room. In her hand, a Shasta daisy. One of those gloriously vibrant, strong blooms nearly bursting with vitality. She asked the members of the group to imagine that this flower represented their life and that each petal was something they were grateful for, something that made their lives rewarding, meaningful, and fun. They were asked to write their thoughts on a piece of paper and share it with the person beside them. Then the nurse made a master list of the "petals" on a flip chart. After doing the exercise, the entire mood of the room was elevated. Counting one's blessings is energizing and fun.

Then the nurse asked the question, "What will happen to these beautiful petals, one by one, as you get old?" She went over to the flip chart and pointed to the first item on the list. "What will happen to our friends and loved ones?" she asked. "They will die." And she pulled out some petals from the flower in her hand and let them flutter to the table in front of her. "What will happen to our health? It will fail." More petals fell. She went through the list: job, home, care, recreation, shopping, eating, reading, traveling, crafts, helping others, independence, etc. The petals kept falling. Soon there was a profusion of disconnected petals on the table. In the nurse's hand was a forlorn stem with a few lonely petals remaining.

The nurse then brought everybody's imagination to the point. Holding up the pitiful remains of that beautiful flower she said, "This is what is happening to our elderly patients. Their lives were once just like our lives: flowers in full bloom. They had all these lovely things in their lives too. Think of the losses they have suffered. Think of all they have had to bear in giving up their petals one by one, or some forced to lose them all at once such as when they have a stroke. When my life looks like this sad flower, I wonder what kind of person I will be. I hope I am cheerful and cooperative and friendly to everyone around me. But I have a feeling there will be days when I don't care about doing what my nurses want me to do. There will probably be times when I will be grumpy and depressed and angry. I may not respond the way others wish I would. I might think they don't understand because, look at them, they're all in the prime of life. Their flowers are full. They have no idea."

The nurse looked over the group and said, "When I think of this flower and my life, I do have an idea. Although I haven't walked in their shoes, I can imagine what they are going through, and I feel so fortunate to be an important part of their lives even when they're difficult." As Fred later shared, "Aura shared this experience over dinner nearly 30 years ago, and it is still vivid in my mind. Our little family did the exercise together at the table. As we did, I thought about an old aunt I had stopped visiting in the nursing home because she was so crabby. That weekend, and many more, we went to see her, and I have never looked at an elderly person the same way since."

This is the power of the imagination to motivate! We can be threatened or bribed into treating people with respect. Think of the push of the regulatory processes such as HCAHPS to make us do what is being measured and monitored. While the behaviors promoted by HCAHPS are valuable and good, the motivation comes from a sense of compliance. Think of strategies we use to reward good behaviors among associates, such as gift cards or a premium parking spot. Again, the behaviors are good, but the motivation could primarily be for the unrelated gain. Another strategy includes having value statements on the wall to keep the concepts front of mind and encourage us to be kind and loving even when we don't feel like it. All of these strategies have their place, can be effective, and may lead to authentic care, but the nurse with the Shasta daisy demonstrates the power of motivating by engaging an individual's imagination. Imagination influences feelings and feelings are the wellspring of desire. When we desire to do something from the depths of this well, it makes our actions easy and natural and real. When we desire to do something, we are *Heartwired*.

COMPASSION + EMPATHY = *HEARTWIRED*

We believe being *Heartwired* is to provide fully compassionate and empathetic care. We also believe being *Heartwired* is a critical component of the "patient-centered toolkit" for anyone working in healthcare today. On the battlefront against disease, associates who are *Heartwired* naturally deploy their compassion and empathy as a force-multiplier connecting two people, once strangers, as newly co-dependent teammates pulling for the same therapeutic win-win. Increasingly evident however is the unwitting disconnect we've created with our sterile, time-sensitive, and technologically advanced workflows and processes so vaulted across healthcare today.

NO TIME FOR COMPASSION?

"Looking back, I realize that in a high-volume setting, the high-pressure atmosphere tends to stifle a caregiver's inherent compassion and humanity. But the briefest pause in the frenetic pace can bring out the best in a caregiver and do much for a terrified patient."

~ Kenneth B. Schwartz, "A Patient's Story"
The Boston Globe Magazine, July 16, 1995

At a time when our abilities to heal, repair, and cure are greater than ever, the satisfaction with healthcare, and in particular the healthcare "system," is lower than ever. In their bold and visionary book called *Compassionomics*, Drs. Stephan Trzeciak and Anthony Mazzarelli thoroughly analyze the role of compassion within modern American healthcare.[21] Spoiler alert: Chapter 1 is entitled "The Compassion Crisis." A survey from Harvard Medical School published in *Health Affairs* asked 1,300 American patients and physicians the question, "Is the US healthcare system compassionate?" About half of patients said the US healthcare system is not compassionate. About half of the patients surveyed also said physicians were not compassionate, while physicians themselves said three-fourths of their colleagues were compassionate.[22] In a follow up to this original study, physicians were asked about their general perception of compassion within healthcare over the past five years. A whopping 63 percent of the physicians surveyed felt they'd witnessed a decline of compassionate care over the past five years.[23] Time to admit the emperor has no clothes. And once we admit the problem, the solution isn't far away.

Must we really leave compassion behind to make budget? Absolutely not! In *Compassionomics* the authors completed a rigorous review of existing research and found quite the contrary. With benefits ranging from happier patients, improved HCAHPS scores, healthier patients, and reduced readmissions, it quite literally pays to be compassionate. In Chapter 9 we will discuss evidence of benefits gained when a healthcare system is full of *Heartwired* providers infusing all they do with compassion and empathy. Leaders would be wise to follow the evidence and work to build compassion in their systems.

Shortly after *If Disney Ran Your Hospital* was published, Fred received an email from Janie Kofford Ford, RN, MS, CFRN, a flight nurse for the University of Utah's AirMed in Salt Lake City. Below is an excerpt from an article she wrote for *Air Medical Journal* that included part of her conversation with Fred:

I'll Take Passion for $1,000

Recently a healthcare institution implemented a new uniform policy based on input from patient surveys. It had been determined that patients perceived nurses in white uniforms as more professional, so the nurses now wear white tops in most areas of the hospital, including the emergency department. Often hospital lobbies more closely resemble a luxury hotel. Name tags are getting longer and longer as more certifications and degrees become the norm, hospital rooms more closely resemble more casual and less aseptic settings; yet when I evaluate the success or failure of a patient interaction, I never consider the uniform, certifications, or ambiance. Rather, I think I am like most patients in that our judgment is based on the way we feel.

What goes into making patients feel that the care they received was exceptional? I like to think of that intangible ingredient as being a passion for delivering exceptional care. Many people have a passion for getting more education or promoting within an organization, but the type of passion that patients actually feel involves that touchy-feely word compassion. What happens in a caregiver's life to obliterate compassion? Conversely, what happens in a caregiver's life to spark compassion? In my own life, it has been a lifetime of health challenges that had me on the receiving end and years of watching the devastating effects of illnesses and accidents on patients' families and trying to somehow make a small impact on that experience.

At a conference, I posed this question to Fred Lee. He is one of the early pioneers of embracing the idea of exceptional patient and customer experiences. His healthcare background was taken to a new level while working for the Disney corporation, and his simple yet profound wisdom can be found in his book. Here, in his words, is the genesis of his compassion-based philosophy:

> "My [first] wife died from encephalitis carried by mosquitoes when we lived in Singapore. She was not yet 29 years old and left behind a two-year-old son and five-year-old daughter. Her physician, who treated her as if she were his own daughter, flew with her on our Pan American World Airways flight all the way to the United States. We had to buy nine airplane seats for her so they could put a stretcher on the backs of three rows of seats. Her physician stood over her the whole flight, responding to every change in her condition. Shortly after take-off the pilot's voice came over the speakers and said, 'Ladies and gentlemen, I am sure you have noticed that we have a critical patient aboard our aircraft today. She does not have anything that is contagious to other passengers. Her physician is attending to her, and if he says it is necessary, we will turn this plane around and fly her back to Tokyo. Thank you very much for your understanding.'
>
> And so I watched anxiously as her physician stood like an angel, bent over her, hour after interminable hour, with a homemade suction device for her tracheotomy and his stethoscope, constantly monitoring, constantly suctioning her, constantly wiping her forehead. When he finally delivered her to the ICU of a hospital in Los Angeles, I followed him into the elevator, and we both broke down and sobbed, hugging each other tightly. I am sure this tragedy and the example of this physician had a lifelong impact on me and the lens through which I see the interconnectedness of all human beings, our fragility, and the importance of how we respond to each other's emotional pain."

We must never underestimate what an overwhelming and emotionally exacting experience critical care transports are for patients and family members. Many areas of medicine have turned their focus to patient-centered input for defining best practices. It is about time! With end-of-life literature replete with descriptions of a "good death," we have to ask ourselves: What is the patient's definition of a "good transport?" Do the phrases "stood over her, responding to every change in her condition," "anxiously... stood like an angel, bent over her, hour after interminable hour," "constantly wiping her forehead," or "hugging each other tightly" come close to describing your practice?

Fred's ability to describe this experience in detail some thirty years later reinforces the power of his feelings of that day. His life's work has been dedicated to making sure that patients and their families have experiences that they, too, can feel and recount decades later. Inevitably, patients and families will scarcely remember many details, but their descriptions will be strong on feelings and emotions. As transport professionals, we play a huge role in the quality of those memories, and, in a sense, we contribute or detract from the healing process that these families experience. If they had only one word to sum up the totality of their experience with us, what would it be? *Efficient? Professional? Competent?* I'll take *compassionate* any day of the week.[24] (Reprinted with Permission)

Most of us seek skill and competence in our healthcare providers. But think about your favorite physician, nurse, physical therapist, or pharmacist. Do you value them only for their skill? More than likely what makes them truly exceptional in your mind is how they make you feel. You are probably quite confident they care about you as an individual, not merely as the patient in Room 201. This sets the stage for you to believe they are clinically competent *and* you feel good about their care. As we have learned, that leads to improved outcomes for you. Your relationship with them is a mutually positive force. They have a passion for their role as healer, and their care for you comes with a large dose of compassion and empathy. We call this a *Heartwired* win-win!

Let's now look a bit more closely at these two key components of being *Heartwired*.

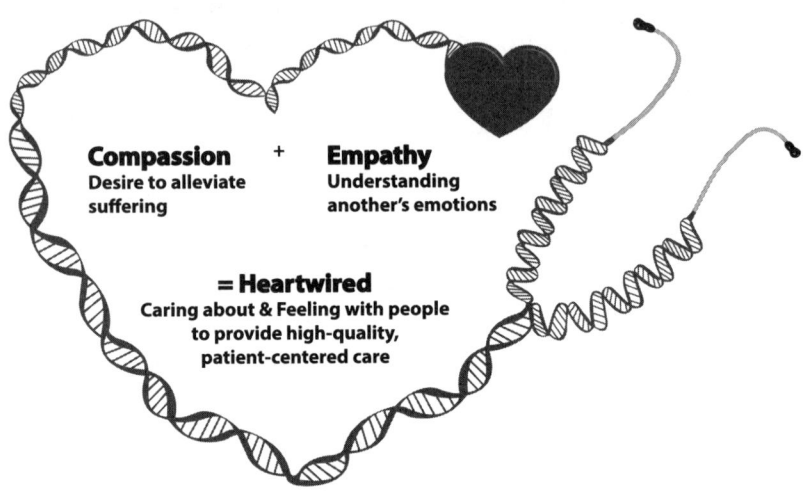

Care and Compassion

"One of the essential qualities of the clinician is interest in humanity, for the secret of the care of the patient is in caring for the patient."
~ Dr. Francis Peabody in "The Care of the Patient."
The Journal of the American Medical Association, 1927.[25]

Historically, medical education has followed an apprenticeship model where students work alongside more senior practitioners and learn the trade as well as the professional standards of behavior. Without question, the most influential of all physicians in the development of modern western medical care in the United States was a physician named Sir William Osler. He lived from 1849 to 1919 and achieved greatness even during a time before antibiotics, modern pharmacologic agents, and specialty surgical procedures were available. Indeed, most of patients could not be cured of their ailments and even he succumbed to an infectious disease now treatable and curable.[26] How is it he was, and in many circles still is, considered "The Great Physician" when he practiced during such a therapeutically impotent time for medicine?

In his article, "Healing and Heroism," H. Brownell Wheeler, MD, provides an explanation:

> "Osler's place in history does not rest on his skill in diagnosis or his effectiveness in treatment. It rests on his profound embodiment of the role of the healer. Osler described medicine as an art, albeit one based on science, and he mastered the art of medicine as few have ever done. He knew that patients are unique individuals and that often their illnesses develop from the fabric of their lives. By adroit and good-natured questioning, he could skillfully perceive the person, as well as the disease. He had a genius at establishing friendships with his patients, in part because he had a genuine and deep interest in them. He could comfort and inspire patients and give them confidence in their ability to get well."

From this standard set by Dr. Osler to modern-day practice, there remains a shared set of professional values. These days most medical school graduations include recitation of shared principles; This first public statement of intent to be of service to fellow man and fellow physicians identifies the expected ethical standards of the professional society. In many schools, the ancient Hippocratic Oath is declared. As with many long-standing traditions, however, there has been a push toward modernizing the text. A current popular version was penned in 1964 by Dr. Louis Lasagna, then Academic Dean of the School of Medicine at Tufts University. His take on the oath for modern times is relevant to our discussion as he chose to infuse it with several key statements supporting the pivotal role of compassion within a healing relationship.

> *"I will remember that there is art to medicine as well as science, and that warmth, sympathy, and understanding may outweigh the surgeon's knife or the chemist's drug.*
>
> *I will remember that I do not treat a fever chart, a cancerous growth, but a sick human being, whose illness may affect the person's family*

and economic stability. My responsibility includes these related problems, if I am to care adequately for the sick."[27]

Among nurses, the origin and legacy of nursing as a profession steeped in compassion is clear from the life and efforts of Florence Nightingale. Much like Osler, she was the embodiment of a life lived for others with a combined ability to care and cure. Nightingale became known as the "Lady with the Lamp" for her nighttime rounds checking on the soldiers' well-being, and ensuring none were left alone in their suffering. Her contributions to organized healthcare are far broader. She was probably the first "Chief Operating Officer" in healthcare as historical details describe that she quite capably took charge of everything from nursing care to dietary services to the plan for sewage management. All efforts were collectively improving the outcomes of the patients, with care and—when possible—a cure. Following these tenets would leave any healthcare provider in excellent standing on HCAHPS ratings. Still, the reality is that few patients perceive such high rates of compassion from their providers (recall the Harvard Medical School surveys we discussed earlier in this chapter). A physician colleague relayed the following story highlighting this distressing fact.

RUTH AND "THE BAD MAN"

Dr. Dean led an outpatient clinic for patients who have concerns about cognitive changes. The most common chief complaint (main reason for the visit) expressed by patients or worried family members was memory loss. One new patient appointment led him to meet Ruth and her devoted husband of many years. As Dr. Dean explained, Ruth was the definition of charm and grace. Well-groomed, articulate, and friendly, it wasn't obvious in the typical social banter of the visit that there was anything amiss. As the evaluation proceeded, however, Dr. Dean came to realize Ruth was having considerable cognitive changes suggesting an emerging dementia.

Ruth described changes to her thinking that had started slowly and infrequently at first. Eventually her husband had noticed and became a terrific support to her making the slips less obvious to anyone else. But eventually it couldn't be denied. Her work as an administrative assistant to a school principal was suffering. A consultation with a local neurologist was arranged. Dr. Dean then learned about "the bad man." As Ruth proceeded to describe her consultation with the neurologist, her tone and demeanor visibly changed. Her spouse quietly watched and listened. As the story progressed it became clear he'd heard this story before but had no intention of trying to change it or his wife's retelling of it. Her words came clearly and intently as she recalled the moment the doctor told her "just like that, she had Alzheimer's disease and she might as well quit her job and plan her funeral." His name was not in her memory but the moniker "the bad man" was. It was clear she knew who she was speaking of even if she didn't remember his name.

Ruth went on to describe the medication prescribed for her by "the bad man." When a possible side effect set in after several days of the medication, Ruth phoned the office for advice. She never received a return call and promptly stopped the medication. She asked Dr. Dean if he would help instead, as she wanted to never return to "the bad man."

Dr. Dean completed the consultation and evaluation. Sadly, he concurred with the original diagnosis and early stage Alzheimer's disease was likely. In the first appointment, no further mention was made to Ruth of a formal diagnosis, but a plan to work together to keep her brain as healthy as possible emerged. Ruth enthusiastically planned a routine of physical and cognitive exercises she would start. Ruth's husband did have a few private moments with Dr. Dean and a social worker on the team. During that conversation, the high likelihood of Alzheimer's disease was discussed and advice given to gently discuss the diagnosis with Ruth if and when she asked for the information in the future.

Over the next year, Dr. Dean saw Ruth and her husband several times. The advance of Alzheimer's was evident in her conversation. She increasingly turned to her husband to fill in details once easily managed on her own. The one area that never waned, however, was her disdain and full retelling of her encounter with "the bad man." How tragic that a person losing precious memories has such a harsh memory still haunting her.

The story of Ruth and "the bad man" serves as a clear reminder that healthcare involves more than prescriptions and procedures. Our words, facial expressions, and attitudes are conveyed to patients and matter to them. Never underestimate how powerful your words are and use them as often as possible as a power to build up and not tear down those you are asked to care for. Perhaps the physician was running behind in clinic and truly didn't want to keep patients waiting. His poor choice of words or lack of tact might have been due to how meticulously "put together" Ruth appeared. Maybe he thought she looked like someone who wanted him to "tell it like it is" and could handle anything. Maybe he was frustrated by a personal disappointment. Or perhaps staff had just complained to him that they were going to have to attend yet another town hall meeting to talk about issues in the healthcare system. Each of us has a myriad of circumstances we face in our daily work as healthcare providers, but the onus is on us to temper those pressures and, in fact, banish them from the encounters we have with patients. No matter the physician's pressures, and even if they rivaled being told you were in the early stages of Alzheimer's disease, if you are on duty your patient deserves your care and compassion.

These conflicting pressures affect everyone working in healthcare. We are all on duty for others but living our own stressful lives as well. Next time you prepare to greet a patient or enter a room, try this: Take a moment to center yourself to the task at hand. You might even use a bit of operant conditioning and teach yourself to focus your thoughts by silently asking "How can I help this patient?" just before you knock or enter the room to greet the next patient. Ours is a privileged profession and patients deserve our focused and compassionate attention to their needs.

The challenge of ensuring healthcare professionals are at once clinically competent and compassionate is not a new conundrum. In 1927, renowned physician educator, Dr. Francis Peabody, penned a seminal essay on the role of compassion as a key professional attribute and skill necessary in the education of physicians. Certainly, his prophetic words still stand for physicians and all engaged in healthcare today.

> The treatment of a disease may be entirely impersonal; the care of a patient must be completely personal. The significance of the intimate personal relationship between physician and patient cannot be too strongly emphasized, for in an extraordinarily

large number of cases both diagnosis and treatment are directly dependent on it, and the failure of the young physician to establish this relationship accounts for much of his ineffectiveness in the care of patients.[28]

Dr. Peabody was prescient in his identification of the role of the physician-patient relationship in the healing process. We learned about that in detail in Chapter 6. Now, let's continue to think of the place compassion holds in the professional tool-kit. In our modern times with the value-based demand that care be both effective and efficient, where does compassion fit? An increasing chorus of professionals and patients alike are asking that it be the foundation of all care.

If Disney Ran Your Hospital was an introduction to the idea that making human connections and showing compassion are key ingredients in quality care. Fred's personal story we shared earlier is a clear example, and the *9½ Things* he wrote about started the movement to transform the healthcare workforce. But even Fred knew merging rich interpersonal interactions in the increasingly fast-paced, economically demanding, and emotionally charged setting of healthcare is not easy. Notable among those working to see such development is the author and healthcare quality pioneer we mentioned earlier, Quint Studer. In his book *Hardwiring Excellence*, one finds an operational strategy designed to foster the development of an organization with a culture of excellence, and compassion. In what seems the perfect end to this critically important lesson, Studer concludes with a personal story involving his brother and sister-in-law. Despite having to endure the unfathomable tragedy of being told by an emergency department team that their 19-year-old son had died in a car accident, months later what they remembered was the kindness of the team involved in delivering the news. Such combined compassion and skill is the high ideal we should all aspire to, leaving patients and families feeling truly cared about. Perhaps fittingly, another offering from the Studer Group, is the groundbreaking work we discussed earlier, *Compassionomics* by Drs. Stephen Trzeciak and Anthony Mazzarelli. Sub-titled *The Revolutionary Scientific Evidence that Caring Makes a Difference*, the authors present a compelling and evidence-based analysis of various lines of research focused on evaluating the role of compassion in healthcare delivery. It's no exaggeration to say the evidence is CLEAR—providing care with compassion makes sense for all involved, the patient, the healthcare providers, and the healthcare systems.

Next stop on our path to being *Heartwired*? Take the foundation of compassion and add empathy.

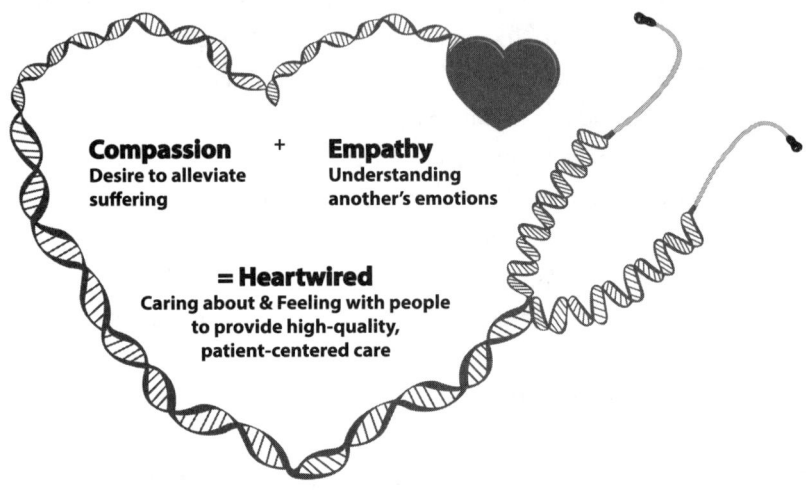

THE EMERGENCE OF EMPATHY

Empathy is "feeling with people."
~ Brené Brown

Compassion, caring, comforting, and kindness—which make up the bulk of adjectives linked to patient loyalty—are rooted in one's capacity for empathy. Is empathy valued by healthcare consumers more than we realize? A 2014 study of 112 patients presenting to Massachusetts General Hand Surgeons suggests it makes up 65 percent of the perceived satisfaction. "Patient-rated physician empathy correlated strongly with the degree of overall satisfaction with the provider. After controlling for confounding effects, greater empathy was independently associated with patient satisfaction, and it alone accounted for 65 percent of the variation in satisfaction scores. Older patient age was also associated with satisfaction. There were no differences between satisfied and dissatisfied patients with regard to waiting time in the office, duration of the appointment, time from booking until the appointment, and health literacy."[29] We believe it is prime time for healthcare to take a truly "patient-centered" and empathetic focus. In 2014 Aubrey Hill wrote in *Health Affairs* about the pivotal role healthcare providers play in a healing process. "Healthcare providers have a unique opportunity to improve patient health outcomes by practicing empathy for their patients and complex life circumstances. Empathy is defined as, 'the ability to understand and share the feelings of another,' and studies have shown that empathy is an important skill for healthcare providers and is significantly associated with improved clinical outcomes."[30] [31]

According to *Webster's New World Dictionary*, empathy is "the ability to share in another's emotions, thoughts, or feelings." It is composed of two Greek words that mean "affection" and "feeling." When people receive our empathy, they feel loved and cared about. In other words, they sense our compassion. "The Daisy Story" uses the power of the imagination to have us "stand in someone else's shoes" and come to understand the role of compassion and empathy in our caring. Teaching and training about empathy can be the catalyst of change across every job category and clinical department in healthcare. By promoting empathy, we can return healthcare to its intended focus of doing no harm and healing with compassion. Who will benefit from this change? We all will. Patients and their families will surely be happier with the care that is high-quality and delivered with compassion. Providers will gain increased personal satisfaction toward their professional calling with less burnout and stress. And healthcare systems will find improved performance across the grading scales with the increased rewards of value-based (not merely performance or volume-based) reimbursements. Believe it or not, all of this can be learned from "The Daisy Story."

Where does empathy come from? It is a uniquely human attribute, not universally present among other members of the animal kingdom. So why did human evolution include the development of this ability? How did we end up an empathetic species? Writing for *Psychology Today*, Rick Hanson, PhD, psychologist and Senior Fellow of the Greater Good Science Center at UC Berkeley, answers the question "How Did Humans Become Empathic?"

> More than learning how to use tools, more than being successful at violence, more than adapting to moving out of the forest into

the grasslands of Africa, it was the complexities of relationships that drove human evolution! *Homo sapiens* means clever ape. We are clever to be sure, but we are clever in order to relate. It would be perhaps more accurate to call our species *Homo sociabilis*, the sociable ape. As Charles Darwin wrote: "All sentient beings developed through natural selection in such a way that pleasant sensations serve as their guide, and especially the pleasure derived from sociability and from loving our families."[32]

Turns out Darwin may have been the first to utter the oft-used saying, "it takes a village!" As Dr. Hanson summarizes "sociability, and empathy at the heart of it, drove evolution…" Our ancestors identified and benefitted from survival benefits when loving families *and* social supports were available to care for each other. Empathy was needed to foster those positive relationships that led to increasingly adaptable and ultimately successful societies. Fast forward to modern-day healthcare and the evidence of benefit from empathy and increased social supports continues to build as models of value-based care become the expected norm. Let's look a bit more carefully at empathy and how it impacts healthcare delivery.

First appearing in *Webster's Dictionary* in 1909, "empathy" is in resurgence and a topic of much discussion as a pivotally necessary and active component of a quality healthcare encounter. Given how valuable we are learning empathy to be, it's reassuring that it is now in the top one percent of lookups on the *Merriam-Webster's* online dictionary and currently in the top ten most searched words of all time. Let's hope many of those seeking to learn its definition are working in healthcare!

Here's how empathy is defined and distinguished from its common companion term, compassion, and from the term sympathy with which it is most often confused. Each of these terms defines a type of interpersonal relationship between provider and patient, yet each has distinct meanings and implications for both parties.

Compassion (Noun): *An understanding* of another's pain **and** the *desire to somehow mitigate* that pain.

Empathy (Noun): The *action of understanding*, being aware of, being sensitive to, and vicariously experiencing the feelings, thoughts, and experience of another of either the past or present without having the feelings, thoughts, and experience fully communicated in an objectively *explicit* manner;

Examples:

He felt great *empathy* with/for/toward the poor.

His months spent researching prison life gave him greater *empathy* toward/for convicts.

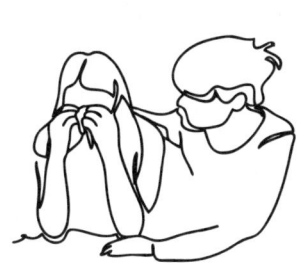

EMPATHY-NOUN

1. The action of understanding, being aware of, being sensitive to, and vicariously experiencing the feelings, thoughts, and experience of another of either the past or present without having the feelings, thoughts, and experience fully communicated in an objectively explicit manner; also : the capacity for this

- He felt great empathy with/for/toward the poor.
- His months spent researching prison life gave him greater empathy towards/for convicts.

COMPASSION-NOUN

Compassion is the broader word: it refers to both an understanding of another's pain and the desire to somehow mitigate that pain:

So empathy is the feeling of knowing someone's feelings, thoughts, or experience while compassion refers to both a feeling *and* the action to do something to in support of the person that stems from that feeling.

Sympathy (Noun): An emotional response by one person to the suffering of another person.

Given the deep interpersonal nature of clinical medicine, it would be ideal for us to know which interpersonal skill, i.e., compassion, empathy, or sympathy, has the greatest potential to create a positive relationship for both patient and healer. While sympathy seems kind, a deeper look reveals it is an emotional response in ourselves to the suffering of others. David Jeffrey, Honorary Lecturer in Palliative Medicine from The University of Edinburgh, writing in *The Journal of the Royal Society of Medicine* describes sympathy as "self-oriented" in contrast to compassion and empathy that are decidedly "other-oriented." This would make sympathy more "provider-centric" so to speak and increases the chance of a provider being personally overburdened. Worse yet, there is no emotional or intellectual connection with the experience of the other person or their emotions per se leaving a gap between healer and patient that has been shown to have negative effects.[33] We are coming to understand clinical medicine needs richer and specifically interpersonal relationships to create bonds of healing.

As we come to know the important role empathy holds in creating effective healing relationships, how does that square with the long-held belief that healthcare personnel need to practice with "detached concern" lest they themselves succumb to their own emotional distress. In such an example, one might recognize that a patient was anxious or depressed but would make no attempt to engage the patient around that emotion and would specifically try to avoid any personalization of the emotion. This form of keeping one's professional distance was felt to insulate healthcare workers from the repetitive and relentless barrage of personal emotional trauma a life in medicine presents. What has been found, however, and beautifully elucidated by psychiatrists Drs. Helen Riess and Dr. Jodi Halpern is that empathy is a successful communication tool which enhances numerous aspects of the interpersonal relationship of healing. As stated by Dr. Halpern, "Empathy allows us to find and experience a shared connection but remain objective and 'other-oriented.'"[34] For compassionate individuals who have dedicated their lives to helping others, learning the value of empathy and the skills of being empathetic, are valuable steps toward being *Heartwired*.

Dr. Helen Riess, a Harvard Medical School psychiatrist, is the leading authority on empathy we met earlier. Her work has helped explain the neurobiology of empathy as well as the impact of empathy within clinical medicine. "In the medical profession, empathy has been conceptualized as a communication competency between clinician and patient, in which the practitioner uses various perceptive routes leading to expressions of concern and compassion."[35] Work in this area has further elucidated two main cognitive elements of empathy. The "affective components" allow us to share the feelings of others and the "behavioral components" motivate us to action. Dr. Riess relates how her own patients would come to their visits complaining about how physicians didn't seem to have time for them. "They weren't seen; they weren't heard; they felt like a number. They were making efforts to change their lives and that wasn't recognized by their physicians."

To study the impact of empathy in clinical encounters, skin conduction studies were performed, allowing assessment of patient's biologic responses to interactions with physicians who had high and low levels of empathy. Other studies showed that better patient-physician relationships improved patients' adherence as well as how they clinically feel and respond to treatment. The benefits of empathy-infused healthcare are broad and extend to clinicians, patients, and healthcare systems alike. Dr. Riess' groundbreaking work is the foundation for a program that trains other healthcare providers in the art of empathy. The website Empathetics.com contains more details and resources. We will review some of the recent research into the benefits of empathy later in Chapter 9.

The Cleveland Clinic has led the way in appreciating the value of empathy and the need to increase its presence across healthcare systems. In their now iconic video, titled *Empathy: The Human Connection to Patient Care (https://www.youtube.com/watch?v=cDDWvj_q-o8)* viewed over five million times and counting, viewers see a day-in-the-life montage of various scenes of life, death, and illness across a typical modern healthcare system. The powerful message is revealed through thought bubbles that hover overhead and give viewers a glimpse into the thoughts and emotions of the various patients and caregivers depicted. This "walk in their shoes" production became the visual for a corporate ethos of empathy also evidenced by the system creating the nation's first C-suite level executive responsible for patient experience. Bridget Duffy, MD, served as the nation's first Chief Experience Officer at the Cleveland Clinic starting in July 2007.

Widespread use of chief experience officer roles didn't take hold until after the government mandated higher patient satisfaction and quality, and tied reimbursement to it. No matter the origin, Dr. Duffy's clinically informed and prescient leadership led her to seize the opportunity to leverage corporate-level financing and resources toward breaking down silos and cultivating a broad culture of empathy with a responsibility to providing compassionate care. In particular, Dr. Duffy held Cleveland Clinic leaders to a high level of leadership accountability for the initiative ensuring its strategic position and operational support to allow success. "Before Duffy took on the role of Chief Experience Officer (CXO) at the Cleveland Clinic, she told leadership that it had to be willing to address fundamental problems with the culture and structure of the organization. Hospital Consumer Assessment of Healthcare Providers and Systems (HCAHPS) scores were between 40 and 60 percent, and people came to the Cleveland Clinic for its reputation of clinical excellence while tolerating the poor service that accompanied it. Consequently, she spent nearly three years working with staff to repair broken trust and relationships between physicians and nurses and addressing caregiver burnout."[36] This thoughtful, comprehensive, and strategically sound approach paves a clear path toward developing sustainable change. We hope there are many similar efforts across the country.

Other systems have reported positive outcomes from taking this approach. The website Empathetics.com is based on Dr. Riess' body of research and contains references to studies evaluating the benefits from the presence of empathy in clinical encounters. Multiple studies have shown that empathy positively impacts healthcare outcomes for the patient, clinicians, and the system as a whole.[37]

Patient-centered Outcomes:

- With improved communication, patients who experience empathetic care have better medical outcomes.[38][39][40]
- Empathy has been linked to better concordance with medical advice.[41]
- Diabetic patients treated by empathetic physicians had a significantly lower rate of acute metabolic complications.[42]
- Empathy from providers helps establish trust within patients and leads to improve adherence to care recommendations and overall effectiveness.[43]
- Empathy from providers was found to be related to lowered patient anxiety.[44]
- Patients who receive bad news cope better when physicians are empathetic.[45]

Clinician Outcomes

- Medical professionals who communicate empathetically have higher patient satisfaction ratings.[46]

- Communicating empathetically increases clinician job satisfaction and reduces burnout.[47][48][49]
- Enhanced communication skills lead to improved diagnostic ability.[50]
- Enhanced empathetic care and physician well-being are highly correlated.[51]
- Empathetic clinician communication improves the quality of all interactions with others; patients, their families, colleagues, and loved ones.[52]

Health System Outcomes

- Reduced burnout and turn-over
    - Communicating empathetically increases clinician job satisfaction and reduces burnout. With 43 percent of nurses showing signs of burnout, it is imperative that we equip them with relational skill sets to better communicate with their patients, work well in teams, and have awareness of their own emotional state. Effective nurse communication is key to patient satisfaction in the healthcare system.[53][54][55]
- Increased patient satisfaction
    - Patient-perceived physician empathy significantly influenced patient satisfaction and compliance via the mediating factors of information exchange, perceived expertise, interpersonal trust, and partnership; potential for increased retention, compliance, reduced excessive utilization.[56][57][58]
- Improved system efficiency
    - Potential for increased retention, compliance, reduced excessive utilization.[59]
    - Increased efficiency of visits.[60]
    - Reduce malpractice claims.[61]
    - Empathetic clinician communication improves the quality of all interactions with others; patients, their families, colleagues, and loved ones.[62]

(Adapted from: http://empathetics.com/why-empathy [63])

EMPATHY: Nature or Nurture, or Both?

The evidence in favor of empathy as a vital aspect of quality healthcare is clear. Empathy is a commonly cited component of favorable patient encounters as well as clinical and operational outcomes. If you were in charge of staffing your healthcare system, you'd probably want to have associates who score high in empathy. But how good are we humans at feeling someone else's pain? Can we truly understand someone else's misery or fear? Do these tendencies come preset at birth or can we learn to be empathetic? Fortunately, it is a bit of both. Some people are born with more empathetic abilities, but no matter someone's baseline tendencies, empathy can be learned. Work from Dr. Riess and others in the field show that it is possible to train healthcare workers in the tools of empathy much like other skills of communication and interpersonal interactions.

As an example, think about the current healthcare workforce age, typically in their 20s to 60s. For these workers, it is fairly easy to empathize with a teen anxious about a blood draw, a young adult working through a painful sports injury, a middle-aged person trying to keep diabetes or hypertension in check, and even women and men starting the required preventive healthcare that marks the start of their 50s. Even if they weren't born with high levels of empathy, since they have a shared experience, these workers often can empathize in these situations. Empathy comes most easily when there is a shared experience to draw upon. But imagine this same workforce helping an 85-year-old learn to walk again after a hip fracture. What does the average healthcare worker know of being 85 years old? Usually, very little. What is their shared experience? Nothing.

This creates a challenging "blind spot" for many healthcare workers active today while the baby boomers continue to age. Americans 65 years and older make up the fastest growing segment of the US population, and by the year 2030, all baby boomers will be at least age 65. At that time one of every five citizens will be over age 65.[64] In typical healthcare settings across most of the US, the presence of elders 65 years and older is nearly 50 percent or more on most days. It can be a challenging time in life when reliable physical function and capability is altered. Some of the dysfunction is merely inconvenient, some embarrassing, some is painful, and some can be fully demoralizing.

Having empathy for this stage of life is challenging since most healthcare workers have absolutely no experience being that same age or even close. Lacking that shared experience, it can be difficult to empathize with those 65 and older facing the realities of physical aging and systematic dysfunction, needing to manage multiple illnesses and symptoms, and/or enduring and navigating the social and family changes and multiple losses only a life of maturity accumulates. We must carefully control our urge to think we might know what it would be like, merely sympathize with pity, or even worse dismiss or refuse to see their reality. Instead, we should realize this generational "blind spot" and take every opportunity to learn and develop our emotional intelligence and powers of empathy for this growing group of individuals who need our *Heartwired* care. It will pay dividends for all of us as one generation after the next learns to understand, acknowledge, and respect the combined triumphs and challenges of living the long lives most of us say we want. In a similar way, we can train healthcare providers to be empathetic to the specific needs of all patients including those they may have very little in common with.

Fortunately, there are ways to teach empathy and we can shore up these "blind spots." Researchers have identified key skills in the area of communication, both verbal and non-verbal, that have proven necessary for expressing empathy.

COMMUNICATING WITH COMPASSION AND EMPATHY

VERBAL SKILLS	NON-VERBAL SKILLS
✓ Active Listening	✓ Body Orientation
✓ Transitional Phrases	✓ Eye Contact
✓ Parroting Responses	✓ Head Nods
✓ Paraphrasing	✓ Voice Tone & Vocal Rhythm
✓ Reflection of Feelings	

Like any skill, these take practice. Next time you have a conversation with a co-worker or patient, consider working on one or two of these skills.

Written for nurses, these skills can be adapted for anyone working in healthcare.

Verbal Communication Skills

- Demonstrating Empathy Using Active Listening: The term "active listening" denotes the set of verbal skills, primarily derived from counseling psychology, that a nurse can use to show that he or she is listening attentively and understanding accurately what the patient is experiencing.
- Transitional Phrases: Occasionally saying "Umhm," "I see," "Okay," and "Go on," provides important signals to the patient that the nurse is attentively listening and encourages the patient to continue talking.
- Parroting Response: With a parroting response, the nurse repeats, verbatim, what the patient said. Sometimes, this is said as either an exclamation or with a questioning tone of voice. Be careful not to use this technique excessively as it will tend to inhibit the patient from saying more.
- Paraphrasing: The nurse uses his or her own words to communicate the same meaning of what was just said by the patient. This is one of the two most frequently used verbal strategies for effectively communicating accurate empathy.
- Reflection of Feelings: This technique is the single most powerful verbal response a nurse can make. To do this, the nurse must listen for the emotion being expressed "between the lines" of the patient's words and state that observation back to the patient. Experience has shown that it is often helpful to start with phrases such as "It sounds like you're feeling _____," "I hear you saying that _____," or "You sound _____ (fill in feeling word)."[65]

Non-Verbal Communication Skills

- Body Orientation: Whenever possible, position your body oriented toward the patient;

- Eye Contact: Occasional direct eye contact can often be a key ingredient in making an empathetic connection to a patient;
- Head Nods: This simple, yet powerful, non-verbal action communicates to the patient that the nurse is listening to what the patient is expressing; and
- Voice Tone and Vocal Rhythm: The tonal and rhythmic matching of the nurse's words and mannerisms to the patient's communication style.

Dr. Riess' work included studying the impact of training physicians to interpret changes in their patients' facial expressions. This evidence has helped reveal that humans are capable of learning empathetic communication skills and behaviors to create the therapeutic connectivity and elicit positive responses seen when patients sense empathy.

"The program teaches facial recognition decoding (is it fear? disgust? surprise?) so that physicians can better respond to those critical cues. It also helps physicians see the vulnerable person behind challenging behavior and new strategies to deliver bad news. Six different specialties at Massachusetts General Hospital took the training course and since then it's been extended to video and virtual training to make an even broader impact. In a randomized, controlled trial, results proved that those three hours are incredibly well spent, instantly improving physician interaction and delivering even better results over time."[66]

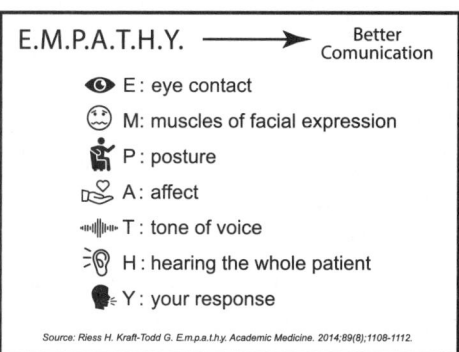

The website Empathetics.com, co-founded by Dr. Riess, contains a full discussion of this topic and includes a review of the evidence base and a range of training tools. A good summary tool is now also available as an interactive app (http://empathetics.com/our-products/) that includes a set of empathy skills training tailored for healthcare associates.[67]

Across many healthcare disciplines training efforts are increasingly focused on developing the skills of empathy and compassion via verbal and non-verbal communication skills. This approach promotes active listening that creates a fuller understanding of our patient's story and the context of their illness. With that foundation, our responses are fueled not with the haste of getting a task completed for the "non-compliant diabetic," but with genuine empathetic motivation to care with compassion. Imagine a nurse admitting a 75-year-old patient with "poorly-controlled" diabetes and pneumonia. With active listening and empathy, we may come to know *and* understand what is fueling the "non-compliance." First, we come to learn the fact that with her failing eyesight due to a combination of aging and diabetes, the print on the auto-injector is now too small for our patient to see. She's been using the injector well for about five years, but diabetic retinopathy and macular degeneration are both advancing. Now, why wouldn't she have simply told her care providers this was happening? We might know the fact, but if we don't know the underlying emotions fueling her behaviors, we won't truly understand her situation. First, she was embarrassed to admit this failing. Second, she was fearful that if she did, someone would say she needed to move to a nursing home. With empathy, we may be able to find a fully compassionate response to avoid embarrassing her and allow her care plan to be adjusted to support this advancing illness and new disability with as much independence and personal dignity as possible. Now imagine you are a busy clinician seeing this patient on her third trip to the emergency department for hypoglycemia. Maybe it's easier not to fully empathize and know her reality? Sadly, that is what happens time and time again to many patients. We can do better and being *Heartwired* is the first step.

Another movement is underway that will support a *Heartwired* workforce toward even greater patient-centered outcomes. Within many models of value-based care are strategies using a team-based approach to care. Imagine if it's not a lone, overworked physician or nurse encountering our 85-year-old who needs an upgrade on her diabetes management; and we aren't calling in an overworked and over-booked social worker to find care despite her lack of funds. As a team of *Heartwired* professionals, we can work together with our full resources of compassion and empathy to understand the realities of our patient's needs and realign her care plan. The medical team will identify her clinical care needs. A social worker will assist by finding out about her family and social network and arranging to get her more support at home. We may work with the low-vision specialists to ensure she has adequate rehabilitative and supportive aids. We can engage her primary care and specialist medical team to begin the challenging conversations about the possible future need for more assistance and the inability to safely remain home. For every patient, their story is the context of their illness and medical needs. By developing our skills of leading with compassion and cultivating our skills of empathy, we will know our patient's story and really know what care they need. That is being *Heartwired*.

COMPASSION IS CONTAGIOUS; COULD *HEARTWIRING* BE TOO?

Like the nature versus nurture debate about empathy, compassion is another basic human personality trait that we are all born with to some degree. It is also modifiable, and highly susceptible to the compassion around us. Has this ever happened to you? You are in the drive-through lane at a fast food restaurant and at the cashier window, the attendant says, "Your meal was paid for by the car ahead of you." Huh?! With a smile and pay-it-forward spirit, you pay for the car behind yours. And so it goes.

Back in the days of the saber-toothed tiger, compassion among humans set the stage for survival; helping each other and relying on the kindness of others helped people stay alive. Our brain recognizes suffering and unfairness, and triggers the "caretaking" center—the vagus nerve—that stimulates a range of actions across the body from our brain to heart and lungs. All designed to help relieve the suffering of others. Undeniably, some of this compassion comes naturally and those who display it can play a key role in inspiring others with their compassion. In her book *Pay it Forward*, author Catherine Rand Hyde introduced the concept of acting kindly at the individual level serving a dual purpose of helping the individual and motivating others to do the same thus creating more kindness in total. As a testament to the value of the creative arts in our human experience, or more simply stated, life imitating art, Ms. Hyde's work of fiction begat a movie which ensconced the term "pay it forward" in our lexicon. The term has come to have two meanings. First, as *the* moniker for contagious kindness, and perhaps more excitingly as a verb for all those random acts one human does for another. The movement is now assisted by a foundation spreading the concepts and compassion globally, (https://www.payitforwardfoundation.org).

As human beings, none of us are perfectly compassionate. We do carry biases that lead us to be more compassionate to some than others. It probably comes as no surprise that we are more likely to help family or friends than a total stranger. We are more likely to help people who remind us of us. Again, there is some evolutionary basis to this, but as time has passed, humans have evolved with wide ethnocultural diversity. Our mandate to be broadly compassionate, especially in the healing professions, is clear. Fortunately, as with empathy, there are ways to learn to be more compassionate. And simply watching others be compassionate can increase our own potential for compassionate behavior. Remember the drive-through lane, compassion is contagious!

The effect of one *Heartwired* associate can be a strong stimulator helping *Heartwire* your whole team. In the popular *National Geographic* series, *Brain Games*, a segment (Season 4, episode 1) on compassion demonstrates this phenomenon. Infants aged 8 to12 months were shown a puppet show in which a cat is seen playing with two dogs. One dog is compassionate when the cat needs help. The other dog is not, and instead acts like a bully. When the infants are later offered both dogs, which do you think they chose? Most infants chose to play with the dog who had shown compassion to the cat. When we see others behaving compassionately researchers believe the hypothalamus releases the "compassion chemical" called oxytocin resulting in feelings of caring, bonding, and empathy. Even better news, engaging in compassionate behavior actually helps create new neural pathways; the more you give, the more you get! Like a pebble dropped in the pond, as more members of the team are *Heartwired* the concentric circles of their positive impact is far-reaching.

In his book, From *Chaos to Care*, Dr. David Lawrence, then CEO of Kaiser Permanente Health System, was an early proponent of the power of team to help improve the care of children with asthma. He describes work done at the Boston Harbor Neighborhood Health Plan through a program called the Community Medical Alliance (CMA):

> Claire Holland is a CMA patient. At 43 years old, she is wheelchair bound with cerebral palsy, a disease that imprisons her normal mind in a body unable to coordinate its movements. Severe spasticity prevents her from walking, her arms flail uncontrollably, especially when she's excited, and she grimaces and sometimes drools down the front of her blouse. But Claire is fortunate in some ways: She can speak well enough to be understood if she remembers to take her time. And she is able to work part time at a small plant that employs disabled men and women two blocks from the group home where she's lived for twenty years, ever since she left her family home after completing City College at the age of twenty-three.
>
> Claire suffers the complications of her chronic illness and the effects of being in a wheelchair: osteoarthritis affects her right shoulder, her hips, and her lower back; she has recurring urinary tract infections from sitting in her wheelchair; and periodically she becomes depressed. She takes several medications each day and receives physical therapy twice a week to relieve the stiffness in her joints and back and the crippling effects of her spasticity. Before she discovered CMA ten years ago, she had great difficulty finding physicians to care for her. When she needed care, she had to find someone to drive her to her physician's appointment, couldn't get on and off an exam table without exhausting herself, and was seen by physicians who had little time to learn about her special needs. So she avoided medical care "like the plague," as she puts it, except for emergencies. As a consequence, she'd never been screened for cervical cancer or breast cancer, she was always running out of medications, and her osteoarthritis

and depression had gotten steadily worse. She was too disabled to work, relying instead on food stamps and welfare to support her limited needs. She rarely ventured out of the group home except to visit her family in south Boston.

The CMA solution for Claire was elegant. The organization enabled her—as it has nearly nine hundred others with severe, chronic conditions—to get medical care within a health plan that serves an overall membership of 135,000 eligible and low-income Medicare and Medicaid individuals. Care is brought to Claire when possible. Professionals teach her how to care for herself; help her caregivers learn medical-care basics that she can't handle alone; and help her arrange transportation, renew her Medicaid eligibility, shop, and take care of personal needs. They also helped her find a job. And they make sure the medical care is accessible and appropriate for her. How is it done?

- Claire and patients like her are full partners in the care process. They are members of the care team.
- Care is provided by a team of providers: nurse care managers, social workers, nurse practitioners, health educators, physical therapists, pharmacists, and, of course, physicians.
- The care process is much broader than the medical care most of us are used to.
- The care teams are nested in an organization that provides infrastructure for the teams to work: information systems, links to community support services, and so on.[68]

Could teams of *Heartwired* associates, patients, and family caregivers be like the pebbles in a pond advancing the quality of care improvements in ever-widening circles across a healthcare system? Would improved care lead to improved patient experience, satisfaction, and health outcomes? Would healthcare systems find improvements in their operations? We believe the answers are, yes. As healthcare quality improvement continues to evolve, value-based care has become the expectation. We believe the successful healthcare system of the future will foster teams of *Heartwired* associates engaged skillfully in the compassionate and empathetic care of people facing illness in their lives.

CHAPTER EIGHT

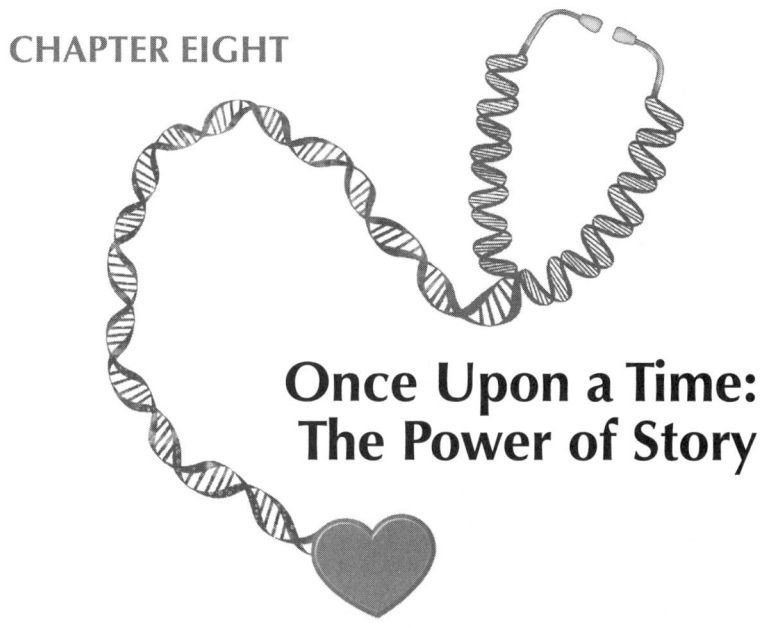

Once Upon a Time: The Power of Story

"In healthcare, making whole again requires knowing the whole."
~ Fred Lee

Our brains are wired to love stories. Our prefrontal cortex, the section of the brain most unique to humans, is abuzz as a story is told and we intellectually and emotionally transport ourselves into the imagined persona, environment, or predicament depicted. Characters in a story we read, hear about, or see up on the big screen come to life in our minds allowing us to "walk in their shoes," relate to their dilemmas, and empathize. In his book, *The Storyteller's Secret*, communications expert Carmine Gallo deconstructs the art and science of storytelling to identify the power within.[69] While the tools of storytelling have evolved from cave pictures to PowerPoint, the utility and potential has remained constant. Stories are our most effective tools of connection and persuasion. Fred's background in marketing led him to understand the potential energy contained in a story. Advertisers know a highly relatable story increases the potential of capturing customers' attention and creating a lasting relationship with their product. Remember the story about the daisy? I bet you do! And I will also bet that story created more than just a memory of the story or a vision of the daisy losing its petals. You probably can quite easily recreate the feeling you got from that story as you came to empathize with the many losses older adults have to face. Researchers have shown that detailed stories can stimulate regions of our brains that would be activated if the event was really happening. Talk about virtual reality! A well-crafted and presented story elicits empathy in the listener and has tremendous power as a tool of connectivity. Earlier we learned of the important role relationships play in creating quality and successful medical care. Could our love of story improve how healthcare providers connect and interact in the time-constrained settings of modern healthcare?

Dr. Rita Charon and others advocating and developing the field of Narrative Medicine believe knowing a patient's story would help all of us, patients and providers alike.[70] In her visionary article, *Narrative Medicine: A Model for Empathy, Reflection, Profession, and Trust*, Dr. Charon describes the field she has envisioned and steered through its formative years:[71]

> Sick people need physicians who can understand their diseases, treat their medical problems, and accompany them through their illness. Despite medicine's recent dazzling technological progress in diagnosing and treating illnesses, physicians sometimes lack the capacity to recognize the plight of their patients, to extend empathy toward those who suffer, and to join honestly and courageously with their patients in their illnesses. A scientifically competent medicine alone cannot help a patient grapple with the loss of health or find meaning in suffering. Along with scientific ability, physicians need the ability to listen to the narratives of the patient, grasp and honor their meanings, and be moved to act on the patient's behalf.[72][73]

She goes on to describe the potential for Narrative Medicine to serve as a guiding model that uses the foundation of the biopsychosocial approach to support a patient-centered and collaborative approach to healthcare:

As a model for medical practice, narrative medicine proposes an ideal of care and provides the conceptual and practical means to strive toward that ideal. Informed by such models as biopsychosocial medicine and patient-centered medicine to look broadly at the patient and the illness, narrative medicine provides the means to understand the personal connections between patient and physician, the meaning of medical practice for the individual physician, physicians' collective profession of their ideals, and medicine's discourse with the society it serves.[74][75] Narrative medicine simultaneously offers physicians the means to improve the effectiveness of their work with patients, themselves, their colleagues, and the public.[76]

The power of Narrative Medicine lies in context. As we learn a patient's story, we understand the full context of this episode of illness in their life. Such context should be a critical factor in determining a care plan but is often completely unknown by treating teams. Consider a retired widower with a new diagnosis of metastatic colon cancer. If you are his physician, which chemotherapy is best? Which will you choose? Before you answer, think about a critical piece of information we are missing. Does he want chemotherapy? Of course he wants chemotherapy, many of us might say. But, in fact, this patient has already had a complicated course of chemotherapy in the past and no longer wants to spend his remaining quality time undergoing medical procedures. Or maybe he's just heard about the toxicity of chemotherapy in general. In either case, in the context of his life, chemotherapy isn't the best answer. He doesn't value treatments that will worsen his life's quality without significantly increasing his survival.

Now consider a patient with multiple sclerosis. If she's a single mother of young children she may balk at the recommendation to take time off work during a disease flare. Her main treatment goals may be to return to work so she can keep her health insurance for her children. An offer of treatment with a medication that can only be administered via intravenous line may be impossible for her to accept. On the other hand, knowing how important it is for her to keep working, her treating team may adjust her care plan to include maintenance therapy that is as aggressive as possible or they may find a way to give her treatment at the end of the day.

Finally, consider an elderly man who is the primary caregiver for his wife who has advanced Alzheimer's disease. He's come to clinic with a binder full of sheets detailing his wife's medications, meals, showers, and bowel movements. He spends what you might consider an inordinate amount of time asking for everyone to review the information. It happens visit after visit and the team begins to loathe their arrival in clinic knowing the data they will need to review. Let's stop and think about what's happening here. Is he a neurotic caregiver? Is it possible he has some dementia himself? Before dismissing him as neurotic, ask yourself, what's his story? In fact, here's his story. The caregiver is terrified his wife will be taken from him if it appears he is an unfit caregiver. Despite being a retired Dean of the Department of Engineering at the local university, he feels woefully unprepared for the role of caregiver to his wife. His detailed descriptions of her daily food intake serve to counter any suggestion that her weight loss is related to his negligence. In the minutes available to a busy healthcare worker, how it is possible to come to know our patient's story? How can we stay patient-centric and quickly learn the context of this episode of illness? We need to stop focusing on *our* stories about them, and learn *their* story.

Before Dr. Charon's work, if someone asked what "narrative" medicine was, most people probably would think it referred to a physician dictating a report of surgery, a history and physical, or a discharge summary, etc. How patient-centered is that?! The main "stories" that fill the charts are provider-directed interpretations and recapitulations of the events of a clinical encounter. The oral traditions of case presentations are similarly told from the provider perspective and embedded with professional speak or jargon shared exclusively among the providers. These practices are geared toward efficient communication among providers with little or no reference to the context of the patient's illness. Here we illustrate just how important context, or story, can be.

Consider this example of a patient brought to an emergency department by emergency response personnel. She resides in a local nursing facility and is alone.

Provider-centered history:

An 87-year-old WW from facility to ED; History of HTN, DM, Dementia. She's combative. Nursing home staff says she was "fine" one day ago, now more confused and not eating/drinking. Full code. No family.

Patient-centered history:

Mrs. Judy Lancaster is a retired RN who suffered a hemorrhagic stroke four years ago and was admitted to the nursing home last year after her spouse and primary caregiver, a retired physician, passed away unexpectedly.

She cannot provide history due to a baseline of dementia and expressive aphasia.

She is fearful when approached and is wary of being touched.

Their only surviving daughter (they lost their only son in military service during Viet Nam), also an RN, lives several states away and has advanced ALS. Her spouse and primary caregiver, the patient's son-in-law, visits when he can and has power of attorney. He's conflicted about end-of-life planning since Mrs. Lancaster is his wife's mother and his wife has not been able to travel to see her. Friends from the local church long attended by the patient and her husband are active visitors and serve as emergency support for the patient/family.

Which "story" is accurate? Both. Which "story" would you want to inform and motivate healthcare providers caring for you? Each of us would want *our* story to be *the* story that sets a foundation for our care. Ideally healthcare providers would know the life story for any patient they care for. Sadly, those "Dr. Marcus Welby" days are gone. While home visits are making a bit of a comeback, the number of people with a long-term relationship with a primary physician or other healthcare provider is decreasing each year. Information exchange about patients is far more likely to be in digital bytes than the human voice. But we can change this. If we take time to learn our patient's story, evidence shows we may be rewarded as sharing patients' stories fires our brains to bring compassion and empathy together in a *Heartwired* therapeutic relationship.

Someday, inevitably, we will be the patient with a story. Empathy is created when we engage on a deeper level of personal, not transactional, knowledge of another person. Living the shared experience of their illness by demonstrating not pity or sympathy but caring and compassion for another human being. In this scenario, Mrs. Lancaster is fully vulnerable and in great need of empathy for her plight. When we learn her full story, we come to have empathy as well for the out-of-town son-in-law beset with unimaginable caregiving duties to both women. What appears to be a forgotten, old, demented lady in a nursing home is quite different. She and her family are in great need of compassionate care to address her care needs appropriately.

In addition to helping healthcare associates provide high-quality and appropriate care, *wanting* to know a patient's story sends a valuable message to the patient that they are more than the gallbladder in Room 304A. They matter. Their story matters to the people who will help care for them. It can be uncomfortable talking about personal matters with perfect strangers. Few patients feel comfortable talking frankly with a physician, nurse, or therapist they've just met. In Veterans Affairs hospitals across the country, the MyLife: MyStory program is underway to ensure the stories of their patients are obtained and uploaded into their electronic medical record for all to read. In the excerpt below the power of story within our human connections is quite clear:

> **FROM the Wall Street Journal July 5, 2019 article "To Improve Care, Veterans Affairs Asks Patients Their Life Stories"**
> Army veteran Fred Lenzen couldn't talk much about the foot he lost in Vietnam; the emotions were still too raw decades later. But he opened up to Mr. Ringler. Once his story was in his record, he said, he felt his military sacrifice was being recognized by the medical staff.

Mr. Lenzen chuckled as he recalled the time a nurse asked him if his foot had been amputated because of diabetes. He told her to read his record. She came back ashen faced, he recalled, and with new respect.

"It makes a difference when they know you from a different perspective than just 'you're a patient here, and we're taking care of you,'" he said, sitting on his hospital bed during treatment for pancreatic cancer.[77]

Just how does such knowing occur? In this case once Mr. Lenzen felt comfortable sharing with a member of the team, his full "story" became known. There had to be that moment of therapeutic trust and alliance allowing him to share. Once that happened, Mr. Lenzen's story was available to all who came to care for him and allowed for additional specific and meaningful connections to occur. In the *Storyteller's Secret*, Gallo shares the research of Dr. Uri Hasson who evaluated the power of story and found how it is that deep and meaningful connections happen from shared stories. In Dr. Hasson's 2010 paper published in *The Journal of Neuroscience*, he presented a novel approach to studying the power of story. He studied both the storyteller and the people listening to the story. Using brain scans called functional magnetic resonance imaging, Hasson discovered that "speaker-listener neural coupling is widespread and extensive." So-called "neural coupling" shows patterns of activity in exactly the same areas of the brain.[78] The sharing of story leads to a connection between the storyteller and the listener that improves the patient experience and adds to the potential of the therapeutic relationship.

Following the publication of *If Disney Ran Your Hospital*, Fred went coast to coast working with healthcare systems on improvements in the patient experience. NorthBay Healthcare in Fairfield, California was one of the stops. In the years following his conference with them, they actively embraced the lessons and created the expectation that patients would be treated as family members with compassion, empathy, and pride. Katie Lydon, RN, MSN, is the Director of Women and Children's Services. In late 2015 she wrote Fred about their ongoing efforts. She shared with him what she learned during a phone call she'd made to a patient who had submitted a poor Press-Ganey survey result. The patient had indicated she was open to being contacted, so Katie took the opportunity. In a memo to her team she shares the story of Jennifer.

> The voice of one young mother who recently delivered her daughter at NorthBay has provided clarity and insight to who we are from the perspective of the patient in the bed. It was in the follow-up phone call I made in response to the lengthy comment she left on the Press Ganey Survey. She left her name and number; it was an invitation for me as the Director to truly listen to her. I am grateful; in fact, I asked her permission to share with others so that they might also hear the voice of a patient and use her experience to truly *connect the work we do* and the tasks on our to-do list *to the memories we are creating for the patient.* That person whose chart we are clicking on in Cerner, the one who we talk *about* maybe more than we talk *to.*
>
> The patient's name is Jennifer and her Press Ganey comments included naming two Physicians that were "absolutely stellar" and two other Physicians who were "completely unprofessional" and who made "inappropriate comments during a procedure." Jennifer wrote that she felt "pushed" by a nurse who "didn't listen to me." She said some nurses were "extremely condescending, disrespectful, and pushy until my test results came back." But Jennifer also named a nurse that was "especially excellent and pivotal in the successful outcome of my delivery."
>
> With this information, I went into the patient record to see who cared for Jennifer during her stay. What came out of the inquiry was a list of "great" nurses—you see, I truly believe that NOBODY comes to work intending to NOT do a great job—yet sometimes we fail to connect our tasks, our med passes, our assessments, the procedures, even the outcomes to a patient's experience—a patient's memory of a life moment. EVERY hospitalization is a

life moment; being a patient is a vulnerable place to be, *our patients TRUST us to provide safe care*, to *care* for them *with competence*, and to *communicate with them, not just about them*.

So, when I got ahold of Jennifer on the phone, I thanked her for taking the time to write the comments, both the good and the bad. I asked her if she could elaborate for me and describe how she felt in the presence of the staff. We started with the *absolutely stellar physicians*. I asked what made her describe them this way. Jennifer said: "Dr. Barling had *exceptional bedside manner*. She was *caring and compassionate*. She *helped me be part of the process*. She was *warm*. Dr. Sarth and I *had a relationship*; she was my Physician in the clinic. She was *clear and compassionate during the stressful process. She told me what to expect.*"

I then asked about what she labeled as *unprofessional and inappropriate* comments during a procedure. Jennifer said: "I felt like the physician was spouting off things. I think she was going over the risks, but the way she was doing it was disconcerting and made me feel awkward and unsure. When she was doing the procedure, she was *talking to the nurse instead of me. Telling the nurse what I should do, like I wasn't able to understand her, almost as if I wasn't there.*"

Jennifer described how she had lost a lot of blood during her delivery and that she felt "extremely dizzy, like I was going to pass out" in the hours after her daughter was born, continuing into the next day. During this time, she said the nurses were "*kind and encouraging, but not listening to me.*" Jennifer felt like the "*nurses were treating me like I was being a dramatic patient, who wouldn't get out of bed. The nurses were cold and pushy about me needing to get out of bed to go to the bathroom. When I requested a bedpan, they seemed irritated and were short with me.*" Jennifer said she "*knew my feelings and that my body was trying to communicate something to me.*" At that point she said,

"I want to talk to a physician." Jennifer described being scared. She was a day and a half postpartum, still dizzy and feeling like something was not right. Labs were drawn, and her H&H had dropped five points since her admission lab work was done. She was transfused two units and "felt like a different person."

One of the cool things that Jennifer offered as she shared her story was that "*L&D nurses did an AMAZING handoff, it was thorough, I felt respected, cared for, and it was healthy.*" She said the "*MBU handoff was not the same, I got the feeling that people were talking about me before they came into the room.*" Jennifer described *the bedside portion seeming more like a "formality, that didn't include me."*

Additionally, when the Pediatrician came in, she got the impression that she was being "treated like a problematic patient," like conversations were happening about her, outside of her presence. In the initial introduction, the Pediatrician talked about how "patients with her personality did this, this, and this…" "How did they know about my personality if they JUST met me? I felt judged because I wouldn't get out of bed due to being dizzy. Like I was being dramatic."

Lastly, I asked Jennifer about the *good nurses*, like the one she described as *especially excellent*. Here are the patient's words as she described the staff who made a difference in her experience: "*She looked into my eyes. She was SO kind. Compassionate. Caring. Present. Informative. Advocate. From the beginning to the end she was a coach at a crucial time. She encouraged me. Great energy. Intentional. Intuitive.*"

I hope you have seen yourself in *this* patient's story. All of our patients have one—a story. We are creating memories for them. Whether they are laying in a NorthBay bed because of a heart attack, knee replacement, sepsis, trauma, stroke, or having a baby, they won't forget the way they were treated and how they felt as they lay in a bed, vulnerable, exposed, and trying to heal.

Don't just punch a clock and complete a task list. Connect. Every patient, Every encounter, Every time.

Katie's phone call to a disappointed patient took a large measure of professionalism including interpersonal tact and humility. How often have problem cases been handled as a "one off" with knee-jerk apology from the CEO and assurances they will get to the bottom of it, only to have it happen again to another, unsuspecting patient and family? Far too often. With a cynical mindset the phone call could be more coldly classified as "service recovery" but within the context of their work to improve the patient experience—notice the name of their program: "Our Shared Stories, Lessons Learned, and Plans to Improve"—it has far more value at North-Bay Healthcare. In the hands of a leader like Katie, this type of program will lead to *Heartwired* associates. Most healthcare associates bring a good deal of compassion to their work. If we create a culture within the workplace that understands the value of a patient's story and the context of illness in their life, compassionate associates will use their skills of empathy to foster therapeutic relationships that add positively to the care of patients.

In his book, *How Doctors Think*, Dr. Jerome Goopman shares his insights about the power of the partnership with patients:

> For three decades practicing as a physician, I looked to traditional sources to assist me in my thinking about my patients: textbooks and medical journals; mentors and colleagues with deeper or more varied clinical experience; students and residents who posed challenging questions. But after writing this book I realized that I can have another vital partner who helps improve my thinking, a partner who may, with a few pertinent and focused questions, protect me from the cascade of cognitive pitfalls that cause misguided care. That partner is present in the moment when flesh-and-blood decision-making occurs. That partner is my patient or her family member or friend who seeks to know

what is in my mind, how I am thinking. And by opening my mind I can more clearly recognize its reach and its limits, its understanding of my patient's physical problems and emotional needs. There is no better way to care for those who need my caring.[79]

Dr. Goopman is *Heartwired*!

The challenge ahead for all of us is to evolve and redesign healthcare from its provider-centric past into a *Heartwired* future. When healthcare is *Heartwired*, patients, family caregivers, and the whole array of healthcare providers care about each other and work together toward high-quality, compassionate, and cost-effective care. Drs. Trzeciak and Mazzarelli of *Compassionomics* provide clear and convincing evidence that caring about people pays off in benefit to patients, providers, and the healthcare system as a whole. We believe *Heartwiring* can help seal the deal and will lead to sustained improvements across healthcare.

SECTION III

THE RETURN ON INVESTMENT (ROI) OF *HEARTWIRING*

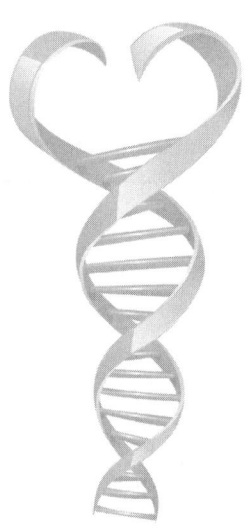

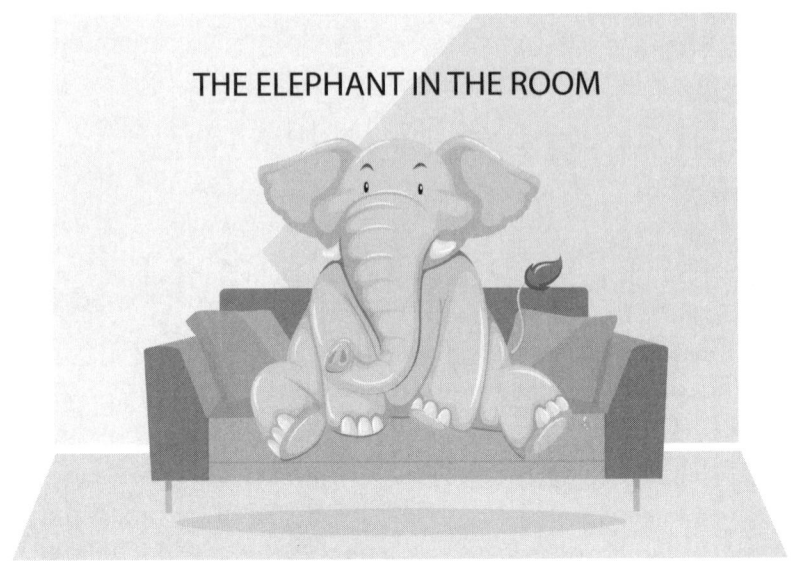

THE ELEPHANT IN THE ROOM

In Section 3 we come face to face with the elephant in the room. Can we afford to be *Heartwired*? Compassion and empathy sound good, but will they support the margin and allow the mission? Sure, an employee at Disney can spend time ensuring satisfaction among their happy vacationers, but this is healthcare where sometimes the news is bad, and we have beds to change over and relative value unit (RVU) targets to meet! Is there really time for compassion and empathy in healthcare? How can we be compassionate, empathetic, clinically competent, and still make budget? *Heartwiring*.

From improving clinical quality, patient outcomes, and satisfaction, we'll explore how *Heartwiring* pays dividends in performance and productivity across a wide range of clinical settings. *Heartwiring* also helps the clinical providers themselves. With compassion fatigue and burnout at record levels, we look at *Heartwiring* as a strategy to provide a valuable tonic for the chronic stress of many healthcare settings. Could *Heartwiring* return some of the joy to healthcare? Can it help with the scourge of burnout, and return skilled associates to full capacity? Healthcare providers will always be under certain stress. Providing medical care will always carry a certain degree of risk. Those we care for will be stressed. But those of us who choose to work in this challenging field are up to the task. Just as technological capabilities are continually improving, we need to continually improve and evolve the human side of caring. Research shows exciting possibility in this area from a deeper understanding of the value of relationships, to evidence that empathy can be taught, to a clear picture of how the human side of healing impacts the bottom-line.

We will push for a new world order that sees healthcare as a team sport with both patient and provider on its roster. Teams caring for and with patients will become the norm in various settings including the hospital (less frequently), a patient's home, outpatient programs, and institutions. Teams will be supported and connected by substantive human connections, supported by modern electronic information and communication methods, and financed by a value-based payment. Teams collaborating to provide compassionate and coordinated high-quality, appropriate and cost-effective care across the healthcare system continuum will be required. *Heartwiring* is the solution.

Our ultimate goal is for every patient to experience the best of what healthcare has to offer from individuals as technically proficient as they are compassionate and empathetic. When a fellow human being is ill, hurt, and suffering, we should lead with compassion and empathy standing as the foundation for the clinical wisdom and technical skills needed to heal. This is what we mean by being *Heartwired*. Many healthcare administrators and clinicians have contacted us after reading the *9½ Things*. They count themselves among those who have gone beyond reading and have adopted the *9½ Things* into their workplace culture. They continue working toward long-lasting and sustainable change. For them *9½ Things* was not just a period of "buzz" about the next best thing in healthcare. They are *Heartwired*.

As more and more healthcare providers become *Heartwired*, the win-win-win of benefits for patients, providers, and the healthcare system will be the norm. In a *Heartwired* hospital, everyone from clinicians, support staff, and administrators alike are guided by genuine compassion and empathy. As *Heartwired* clinicians, the patients we care for are not merely customers but people we know and care about. Their individual stories can be shared as often as their age, gender, major medical diagnoses, and current medications. Our ability to heal is enhanced when we forge genuine human connections along with surgical repairs, intravenous medications, or a course of physical therapy. And patients are not merely satisfied, but die-hard fans, loyal to the system and clinicians who are *Heartwired* toward truly patient-centered care. If there is any *pixie dust* to be had in healthcare, our bet is on *Heartwiring*.

So, let's meet that elephant…

CHAPTER NINE

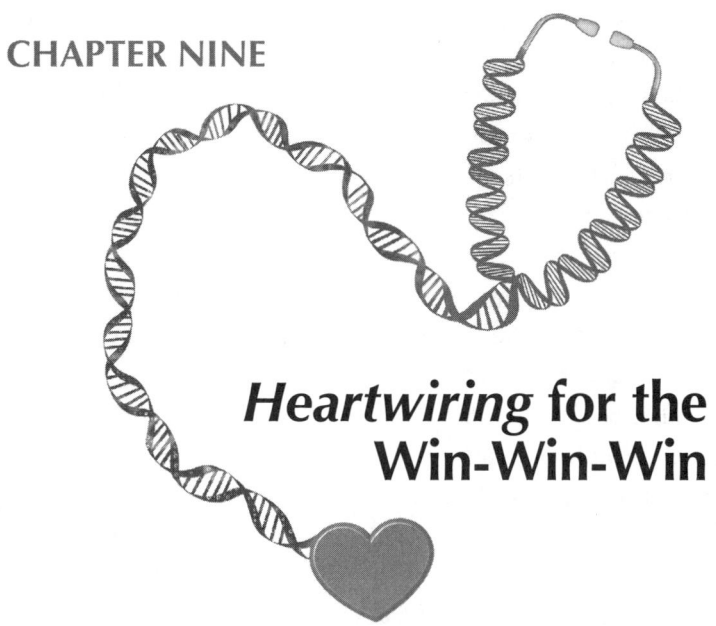

Heartwiring for the Win-Win-Win

"No Margin, No Mission."
~ Sister Irene Kraus
Inaugural President of the Daughters of Charity National Health System
Past Chairman of the American Hospital Association's Board of Trustees.

CAN HEALTHCARE REALLY AFFORD TO BE *HEARTWIRED*?

Imagine you are an advanced practice registered nurse (APRN) working in a primary care clinic. As you approach Room 2, a quick glance at the chart leaves you thinking you will surely get back on time with this easy visit. Mrs. Burns is in clinic for a medication check. She is well known to you and a highly compliant patient. Before you walk in, the medical assistant asks, "Did you hear?" and goes on to tell you that quite unexpectedly Mrs. Burns' only daughter died last week from a ruptured brain aneurysm (abnormal blood vessel in the brain that ruptured and created a fatal brain injury). No, you had not heard this terrible news. Now what? Clearly there is a need to address this sad and devastating loss. But do you actually have time in the schedule to stop, empathize, comfort, *and* check her new blood pressure medication? Of course not. But, of course, you need to devote time for all of that to this patient. Under the circumstances it needs to be done. Later that afternoon, now hopelessly behind schedule, can you summon some compassion and agree to see the patient who arrives twenty minutes late after an accident on the interstate created a traffic delay? Can a hardworking provider actually make the RVU goal, keep all patients on time, well cared for, and satisfied? What about the nurse practitioner herself? Will she leave clinic on time to see her son's soccer game? Were all the charts completed before she left work? Or will she do the chart documentation, yet again, at her dining room table after clearing away the dinner dishes and getting everyone else set for the night. How do we keep the compassionate healthcare coming within a solvent system while infusing it with all we've learned about the power and potential of *Heartwiring*? What will it cost in dollars and human capital to *Heartwire* a healthcare system? Is it worth it? We cannot escape the question, and we argue, we shouldn't. *Of course*, we can only provide care we can afford to provide. If we want something more from healthcare, we will need to do a certain type of work to keep the profit/loss statements balanced. The challenge ahead is to qualitatively evolve the delivery of healthcare, i.e., to *Heartwire* healthcare to include compassion and empathy within a high-quality, satisfying, cost-appropriate and cost-effective system.

As is always the case, we stand on the shoulders of those before us. In Chapter 2 we learned about Deming's seminal work in Total Quality Management. From those lessons we are able to continuously improve the process of caregiving leading to improved quality of care as well as financial performance. Quint Studer's work helped us understand and operationalize sustainable success via Hardwired Excellence.[80] Another Studer Group offering, *Compassionomics*, takes the field forward again by detailing the evidence that shows caring is good for the patient and good for the bottomline. We believe the next evolution needed is to *Heartwire* healthcare. We believe *Heartwiring* is a win-win-win where patients, providers, and our healthcare systems will benefit. Remembering that Compassion + Empathy = *Heartwired*, let's look at some data.

HEARTWIRING HEALTHCARE IS A WIN FOR THE PATIENTS

> *"Treat the disease, you win, you lose; treat the patient, I guarantee you'll always win."*
> ~ Patch Adams, MD

Do patients benefit if they are cared for by a *Heartwired* provider or team? Are they more satisfied? Do they feel they are getting better care? Does it matter to the patient that the physician is *Heartwired*? In Chapters 7 and 8 we discussed a range of benefits that have been seen when compassion and empathy are part of healthcare delivery. Let's look in more detail at the effects of compassion and empathy on patients.

A research group in the Netherlands studied physician-patient interactions by videotaping encounters between 142 Dutch physicians and 1,388 patients. A primary focus was evaluating how physician behavior and communication styles might impact the information an anxious patient would reveal to the physician. Among patients who perceived a more empathetic physician, lower rates of anxiety and improved communication about the patient's concerns were found. The physician's behavior and non-verbal communication played a pivotal role in affecting patients' anxiety levels and allowing patients to fully express concerns.[81] At this point you might be thinking, where's the news here? Isn't that a "no brainer?" Seems obvious that "nice physicians" make patients feel less anxious. True enough. We could stop here with a patient-centered result in favor of physicians being nice. But we are pushing the discussion into the economic arena. Remember: no margin, no mission. If we have a group of really nice healthcare providers but their practices are so inefficient they can't make budget, we lose the benefit to the patient. This research looked further and provides evidence that there is real human *and* economic value of a healthcare provider behaving with compassion and empathy.

The researchers looked deeper at some of the specific differences found in the care provided to patients who had high levels of anxiety and those with lower levels of anxiety. The researchers found that high-anxiety patients asked more often for services like a prescription or referral. While the research did not define why, it could be patients were less inclined to talk with the physician and instead wanted medication or another physician. Consultation time was significantly longer with anxious patients: the average consultation length for low-anxious patients was 9.30 minutes (SD=4.37), for medium-anxious patients: 10.24 minutes (SD=4.80), and for high-anxious patients 11.25 minutes (SD=4.95). Again, while we don't have details explaining why, in this study, physician behavior appears as an active component of the quality and quantity of a healthcare encounter.

How long it might take for a physician to leave a patient feeling less anxious? Let's look at a study designed to answer that very question: "Can forty seconds of compassion reduce patient anxiety?" Researchers used a standardized videotape to assess the effect of physician compassion on viewers' anxiety, information recall, treatment decisions, and assessment of physician characteristics. One hundred twenty-three healthy female breast cancer survivors and eighty-seven women without cancer were recruited for the study. Women who saw an "enhanced compassion" videotape rated the physician as warmer and more caring, sensitive, and compassionate than did women who watched the "standard" videotape. Women who saw the "enhanced compassion" videotape were significantly less anxious after watching it than the women in the other group. Those who saw the "enhanced compassion" videotape rated the physician significantly higher on other positive attributes, such as wanting what was best for the patient and encouraging the patient's questions and involvement in decisions. The authors of the study concluded that the "enhanced compassion" videotape was effective in decreasing viewers' anxiety.[82] Other studies have found similar results with the median value of five studies showing that demonstrating compassion took forty seconds.[83] Only forty seconds. Even briefer interactions can have profound impact. In his book, *Why People Die by Suicide*, psychologist and expert in suicide, Thomas Joiner, tells of a suicide note containing the statement: "If just one person smiles at me on the way to the bridge, I won't jump."[84] A smile takes only one second. Our interactions, no matter how brief, are impactful. As Mother Teresa stated, "We shall never know all the good that a simple smile can do."

This research suggests that a *Heartwired* provider who pays attention to how they communicate and interact with patients can efficiently create a positive therapeutic environment that will lead to visits of higher quality with patient-centric discussions, diagnoses, and care plans. Clearly a better outcome for patients than encounters that end with knee-jerk prescriptions or unnecessary referrals to specialists or testing. Later we present a tool-kit for leaders who wish to see their associates trained in *Heartwiring*. We've seen how our investment in developing *Heartwired* associates and care teams will have a positive ROI for the patient. Could *Heartwiring* prove helpful to the providers themselves?

HEARTWIRING HEALTHCARE IS A WIN FOR PROVIDERS

"If you don't love yourself you cannot love others. You will not be able to love others. If you have no compassion for yourself, you will not be able to have compassion for others."
~ Dalai Lama

Think back to the last time you were on an airplane and the flight attendant was giving the pre-flight instructions. By federal regulation these instructions include the fact that in the event oxygen masks are needed, you should secure your own mask before assisting any children or others around you who may need help. Doesn't immediately seem to fit in a book about compassion does it? It may not seem to be the compassionate choice, but ensuring the capable adult has the ability to be available for others less capable of helping themselves is critically important. This advice turns out to be valuable in day-to-day life as well. In the book *Take Your Oxygen First*, family caregivers of patients with Alzheimer's disease and other memory loss disorders are given this recommendation to ensure they are able to withstand the chronic and daily stresses of providing care support to a loved one with an illness as devastating as they come.[85] Now imagine you are an EMT heading to work but feeling dread because you are burned out. Work has been more demanding due to your partner having been injured, your daughter has had trouble adjusting to her new school, and you just signed up for three extra shifts this month. You didn't take your oxygen mask first. And now you, your family, and the patients may suffer. Healthcare providers face chronic stress in their professional caregiving roles and need to take their oxygen first. By donning that oxygen mask first, they bolster their ability to be compassionate and empathetic and reap the full range of benefits of being *Heartwired*.

We now return to the work of Drs. Trzeciak and Mazzarelli. In their book, *Compassionomics*, they masterfully detail a body of research summarizing the impact of compassion and empathy on the well-being of healthcare professionals and students. Their detailed review of the literature is a complete eye-opener. Conventional wisdom has been that the more compassionate a healthcare provider is the more likely they will burnout from the weight of emotional distress they encounter. It follows that those with low compassion would be less likely to burnout since they would have protected themselves by keeping their emotional distance. Guess what? Conventional wisdom is WRONG! Evidence shows that compassion and burnout go in the *opposite* direction.[86] We will discuss burnout in more detail in Chapter 10. For now, let's continue on and talk about how, in addition to avoiding burnout, being *Heartwired* with compassion and empathy actually leads to positive benefits for healthcare workers.

A study from the Mayo Clinic found that higher rates of compassion and empathy were associated with lower depression symptoms, a higher sense of personal accomplishment, and enhanced quality of life.[87] The concept of compassion satisfaction—or the amount of pleasure one gets from compassion for others—is felt to be at the core of this finding. As Drs. Trzeciak and Mazzarelli state: […] the human connection can transform the experience for the giver of compassion, trigger positive emotion, and build resilience. (That's the ability to maintain one's own well-being despite stressful conditions, including witnessing suffering.)[88]

With all the evidence showing the benefits of compassion and empathy in today's healthcare, it seems reasonable to assume both would be easy to find in physician's offices, emergency departments, and all across healthcare systems. Afterall, aren't people who go into healthcare typically compassionate people? While it is true healthcare attracts people with a disposition to compassion, there are competing factors that often reduce its active presence or—in the worst-case scenario—snuff it out completely. Medical training can be rigorous with long hours spent in relentlessly stressful environments. Patients are complicated. Families are stressed. Resources are finite. The economic realities of making the margins work to support the mission often mean doing more with less. And then there's the electronic medical record. All one has to do is watch the Athena commercial called "When I Grow Up—Athena Health" (search for the video by name on YouTube) to learn of the potential for the electronic medical record to destroy any potential human connection and suck the compassion and empathy right out of the most well-meaning healthcare provider. Fortunately, however, there is good evidence that while compassion and empathy may be on life-support we can bring them back.

Let's start by doing some myth-busting. Sometimes it's erroneous beliefs of the healthcare worker themselves that limits their compassion and empathy.

Common Conventional Wisdom (CW) for being "all business" in healthcare, and the Facts that prove *Heartwiring* is the better way

CW: I am compassionate.
Fact: Maybe, maybe not. You may not be the best judge.
Evidence: Physicians' self-rating of their emotional intelligence did NOT correlate with how patients viewed them. Nurses rating of physician's emotional intelligence DID correlate with how patients viewed the physicians.[89]

CW: Patients want my skill, not my heart.
Fact: Patients don't care how smart you are, they are more impressed if you communicate clearly and treat them well.
Evidence: In a *Wall Street Journal* article, results of a Harris Online Poll reveal what adult consumers value in their healthcare relationships. This data probably only surprises those of us in healthcare. While training matters, it is

illuminating to see the magnitude of difference between the import given to interpersonal skills.

"Which of the following qualities are *extremely important* to you in the physician or physicians who treat you?"

- 85 percent: Treats me with dignity and respect
- 84 percent: Listens carefully and is easy to talk to
- 27 percent: Has been trained in one of the best medical schools[90]

CW: I need to keep my emotional distance.
Fact: Compassion doesn't lead to burnout, it protects against burnout.
Evidence: Refer back to the evidence in Chapter 9,[91] or just remember this, *"If you want others to be happy, practice compassion. If you want to be happy, practice compassion."* ~ Dalai Lama

CW: I don't have time.
Fact: Yes, you do. You have forty seconds and it takes JUST forty seconds.
Evidence: "Even simple self-reminders may reinforce the motivation to be compassionate. Rather than the neutral maxim *'primum non nocere'* or 'First, do no harm', silently repeating 'May I be of benefit' when hand sanitizing, touching a patient, or auscultating is a more proactive approach to daily professional practice."[92]

CW: I am not touchy-feely.
Fact: No problem, there's an app for that! Compassion and empathy are skills that can be learned.
Evidence: The work we referenced earlier from Drs. Kelley and Riess showed that.[93]

We've discussed the benefits of *Heartwiring* for patients and healthcare providers. Let's next think about the potential benefits to the larger healthcare system. With the crisis of ever-escalating healthcare costs, could *Heartwiring* be part of the solution to steady those costs?

HEARTWIRING HEALTHCARE IS A *WIN* FOR HEALTHCARE SYSTEMS

"All that changed on November 7, 1994, when at age forty I was diagnosed with advanced lung cancer. In the months that followed, I was subjected to chemotherapy, radiation, surgery, and news of all kinds, most of it bad. It has been a harrowing experience for me and for my family. And yet, the ordeal has been punctuated by moments of exquisite compassion. I have been the recipient of an extraordinary array of human and humane responses to my plight. These acts of kindness–the simple human touch from my caregivers–have made the unbearable bearable."
~ Kenneth B. Schwartz, "A Patient's Story"
The Boston Globe Magazine, July 16, 1995

Let's look at how *Heartwiring* a healthcare system and increasing acts of kindness that were so affecting for Mr. Schwartz, might have a positive ROI. A patient's story about kindness may seem an unlikely starting point for this discussion about the "business side" of medicine, but in fact it is *the best* starting point. As we've come to understand, context is everything. A patient's story, their experience of interacting with the healthcare system, and the ability of that system to care with compassion, empathy, quality, and cost-effectiveness, are the key factors in the business of healthcare.

A common goal for many healthcare systems is summarized by the Institute for Healthcare Improvement's "Triple Aim" of "improving the health of populations, enhancing the experience of care for individuals, and reducing the per capita cost of healthcare."[94] Simply put the "Triple Aim" strives to improve the health of our communities through healthcare systems capable of providing high-quality, satisfying, and cost-effective care. Could *Heartwiring* healthcare lead to achieving the "Triple Aim"?

YOUR EMPATHY IS SHOWING

Consider the care of patients with diabetes—one of the most common chronic illnesses in the world. It's also an illness with high potential to lead to poor patient outcomes and high healthcare expenditures. A research group tested the hypothesis that physicians' empathy is associated with positive clinical outcomes. They followed 891 diabetic patients over a three-year period and followed their disease management via hemoglobin A1C and LDL-C (cholesterol) levels. Their physicians completed a standardized survey designed to identify empathetic traits and behaviors (Jefferson Scale of Empathy), and were categorized into high-, medium-, and low-empathy categories.[95] Patients of physicians with high-empathy scores were significantly more likely to have good control of hemoglobin A1C and better levels of LDL-C than were the patients whose physicians had low-empathy scores. High empathy = improved diabetes management. Most likely you can change out the condition diabetes and similar findings would be true for a range of chronic illnesses such as congestive heart failure, asthma, and COPD.

Patients whose physicians were high on the empathy scale had better clinical outcomes. They were more satisfied. They rated their providers more highly for care. Providers were more fulfilled. Satisfied patients and fulfilled providers. What is the impact on the healthcare system of happy patients and providers? Costs go down.

In a study that followed 1,824 patients with diabetes over a two-year period, researchers compared 912 patients whose hemoglobin A1C had improved to 912 patients who had not seen hemoglobin A1C improvement. Patients who had improved had average annual healthcare costs that were 24 percent lower during the first year of follow-up and 17 percent lower during the second year of follow-up, compared to patients whose A1C did not improve. This reflected a savings of US $2,503 and US $1,690, respectively. For both time periods, the outpatient category was the largest contributor to cost savings.[96] High physician empathy leads to engaged patients with improved patient outcomes and improved outcomes can reduce healthcare costs.

HAPPY PATIENTS STAY HOME

A group from Cleveland Clinic Joint Arthroplasty published results of a study designed to determine whether readmissions within thirty or ninety days following discharge was associated with HCAHPS scores for total hip arthroplasty patients. Their study of 1,868 patients included 578 patients who completed the survey. Of those a significant negative association was found between readmissions and HCAHPS score dimensions including nurse communication, physician communication, pain management, and global satisfaction with the hospital experience.[97] The moral of this story seems simple enough, but is difficult to achieve. Patients who report high levels of communication with the healthcare team and are highly satisfied with their care will have better outcomes and fewer hospital readmissions. Unhappy patients, on the other hand, are more often readmitted and report lower levels of communication. Finding ways to ensure quality care is achieved with compassion and empathy will pay dividends for both patient and staff.

In both examples, a *Heartwiring* win-win-win *and* Triple-Aim achieved.

As we have said, of course, we can only provide care we can afford to provide. If we want something more from healthcare, we will need to do a certain type of work to keep the profit/loss statements balanced. The challenge ahead is to qualitatively evolve the delivery of healthcare, i.e., to *Heartwire* healthcare, to include compassion and empathy within a high-quality, satisfying, cost-appropriate, and cost-effective system. Next, we describe several strategies to make the shift while keeping in mind the necessary Triple-Aim.

TALK ABOUT IT

Rather than shy away from the difficulties and emotional demands of healthcare and ignore the impacts on healthcare workers, we recommend hospitals or other healthcare operations establish "Schwartz Rounds" to allow a forum for staff of all backgrounds to come together and talk about the emotional and social challenges of caring for patients.

The idea for these interdisciplinary and evidence-based forums came from the extraordinary patient advocate we quoted earlier, Mr. Ken Schwartz, who started the non-profit Schwartz Centre for Compassion in Healthcare prior to his death in 1995. Mr. Schwartz was a seemingly healthy 40-year-old non-smoker when he was diagnosed with advanced lung cancer in the fall of 1994. The following year of medical care and treatment preceding his death were in his words a "harrowing experience" but filled with moments of "exquisite compassion" that made "the unbearable bearable." Amid the devastation of his life's cruel fate, he keenly recognized the damage caused when bad healthcare systems happen to good healthcare workers. He used his limited time to develop the Centre with a mission of promoting kindness and compassion in healthcare workers and to specifically "encourage the sorts of caregiver-patient relationships that made all the difference to him." Today in over 230 sites in the US and abroad, Schwartz Rounds have shown benefit to individuals, teams, and hospital culture. Attendees have been found to have decreased stress and feelings of isolation, a greater understanding and appreciation of colleagues' roles and contributions, and feel more supported in their work and able to provide compassionate care.[98]

IT'S WRITTEN IN THE STARS

Like it or not, ratings of our individual and system performance in healthcare are here to stay. Evidence abounds even back to the days of Deming that what we study, improves. This is true of assembly line processes and human behavior. So, enter the CMS Stars.

Among Medicare Advantage plans, CMS assigns quality via a "Star Program." From the patient/member perspective, the plans are evaluated in these 5 areas:
1. Staying healthy: screening, tests, and vaccines
2. Managing chronic (long-term) conditions
3. Plan responsiveness and care
4. Member complaints, problems getting services, and choosing to leave the plan
5. Health plan customer service

The assumption is that higher-rated programs will perform better for Medicare Beneficiaries. There is some evidence this is the case. One investigator found an association between the CMS Star Program and lower rates of in-hospital complications and lower rates of unplanned 30-day readmissions to the hospital.[99] If you were in charge of the Medicare budget, what would you say? Who would you want to pay for care?

Facing this scrutiny, operating a successful healthcare system will require leaders dedicated to supporting their associates and clinicians with sufficient resources to offer state-of-the-art care and technologies with compassion, empathy, and stellar customer service. It will take the continuous quality improvement we've discussed, and then some. While we believe the discipline of addressing work performance deficiencies with PDSA cycles and measuring for improvement is sound, we also know a healthcare system cannot ignore its unique relationship with the consumer. Our consumer isn't always right. And in some cases, to avoid outright malpractice, we cannot follow a prescribed customer-service script that suspends judgment and—for the sake of avoiding conflict—*pretends* our consumer is right. If we wholly measure performance by HCAHPS or STARS, and even tie ever-increasingly significant percentages of reimbursement to it as is happening today, what's a physician or nurse practitioner to do? Should they give in and write the script for an antibiotic when we really think it's a viral infection? Should they give in and prescribe the narcotic pain medication the patient has now asked for three times? Our consumer isn't always right, but what happens if we make them an unhappy customer? To balance this unique marketplace position, a healthcare system needs a culture of excellence that understands these limitations but still pushes itself forward. The best systems *Heartwire* their culture of excellence to use continuous quality improvement principles while supporting its professional ethos and responsibility to its unique consumer, called patient.

DOES CULTURE EAT STRATEGY FOR LUNCH?

The common business school colloquialism, culture eats strategy for lunch, is now considered conventional wisdom. But does culture in fact change outcomes as directly as a strategic decision might? For example, what's the return on investment for a positive culture among your associates compared to a decision to pursue a new line of business? We've discussed how workplace culture seems to set the stage for associate performance. Recall the strong culture of Disney associates carefully adhering to the rules of etiquette and proper attire. Is the Disney *culture* why Disney outperforms many other companies in customer experience?

In an article published in the *Journal of Healthcare Leadership*, analysts identified a process for measuring relative rates of culture among healthcare systems and then evaluated the impact of workplace culture on a range of economically active factors in healthcare settings.

Culture was measured through self-reported employee feedback surveys:
- The extent to which patients are treated as valued customers
- You find that your values are very similar to the values of this organization
- You feel that being a member of this organization is very rewarding
- You are proud to be part of this organization

Here is how culture impacted certain performance outcomes:[100]

	Top Quartile Culture Index	**Bottom Quartile Culture Index**
Willingness to Recommend:	72	26
Average Earn-Back: (Percent of Value-Based Payments)	2.4%	1.4%
Turnover Rate:	14.7%	17.9%

Did you notice the measured items include some patient-centric items to ensure we have focused on our core activities? And then notice these measures evaluate shared values and ask how associates feel as a member of the organization. Do we share the same values toward our work? Are you feeling rewarded and proud? No more can the focus be only on the patient outcomes (though we'd argue these are *always* included), but should include associate well-being as well. You can't script the nurses to apologize for delays and then have the nurse-patient ratios below standards. Both need to be measured, managed, and improved. According to researchers Barsade and O'Neill, there is a direct connection to how employees feel about their workplace, their level of engagement, and job performance. In their longitudinal study, "*What's Love Got to Do With It?: The Influence of a Culture of Companionate Love in the Long-term Care Setting*," based at a long-term care facility and hospital in the Northeast, the researchers surveyed 185 employees, 108 patients, and 42 family members on two occasions sixteen months apart. The "Love" they were researching is not romantic, but companionate love. The authors explained that companionate love is based on warmth, affection, and connection rather than passion. To really make the point, the authors provided a well-known example of a workplace culture that is strongly influenced by companionate love. Southwest Airlines, famous for its culture of caring and fun as well as flying airplanes, wears its love on its sleeve so to speak. The ticker symbol for Southwest on the New York Stock Exchange? LUV! What the researchers found in their study was that culture did indeed have a strong influence on workplace outcomes. Employees who felt they worked in a loving, caring culture reported higher levels of satisfaction and teamwork, they showed up to work more often, and contributed to improved outcomes for the residents. The study found improved patient mood, quality of life, satisfaction, and fewer trips to the emergency room.[101] Talk about culture eating strategy for lunch!

When you have an alignment of culture like this, you are *Heartwired* for excellence and will have a higher functioning health system with healthier, happier patients and associates.

CHAPTER TEN

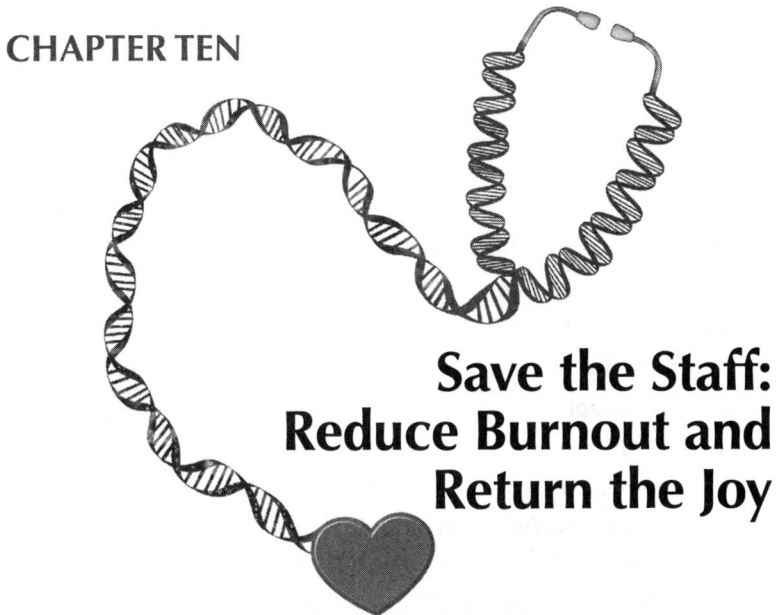

Save the Staff: Reduce Burnout and Return the Joy

"If we don't take care of ourselves, we cannot survive."
~ Dalai Lama, 2016
The Book of Joy: Lasting Happiness in a Complex World

Which Stone Mason are You?
The Story of the Stone Masons

> Once there were two stone masons. As they worked at a building site one day making perfect bricks one after another, each one of them was asked, do you like your job?
>
> The first man answered flatly, "It's a job, it pays the bills." The second man was beaming with pride and declared, "I love my job, I'm building a cathedral."

Which "stone mason" do you want on your team as you work to solve a difficult problem at work? How about as you rush into an emergency trauma call? Which would you like heading into a patient's room to deliver bad news or draw blood? Certainly, not the first stone mason. His detached, task-specific answer smacks of burnout, doesn't it? The second stone mason, now I want him on my team! This man shares a great vision with others as they work together to build a cathedral. He understands his role, and does his work with great pride. His positive attitude is likely to encourage and inspire others.

Our attitude and perspective do indeed make a big difference in how we approach our work. In his terrific book, *Start with Why*, author Simon Sinek, stresses the importance of "starting with why" and allowing that purpose to set the stage for our work. "Starting with why" inspires people to act in a certain way.[102] In healthcare settings, we've talked about how important the therapeutic relationship is to the outcomes for the patients. The attitude and perspective of healthcare providers—their "why"—is a critical requirement in creating authentic and effective therapeutic relationships with patients. Their "why" bolsters their emotional stability with feelings of self-worth and contentment, and fuels mutually positive relationships with colleagues and other associates. If we are waking up each day ready to do our part to "build the cathedral," it's more likely we will thrive personally and professionally amid the diverse challenges of modern healthcare.

BAN BURNOUT

Burnout should be considered enemy #1 to our efforts to *Heartwire* our healthcare systems. As described by leading experts Christina Maslach and Michael Leiter in their 2016 article, there are three core dimensions of the burnout experience:[103]

Exhaustion:	Wearing out, loss of energy, depletion, fatigue
Cynicism:	Negative or inappropriate attitudes toward clients, irritability, withdrawal
Inefficacy:	Reduced productivity or capability, low morale, inability to cope

The demands on healthcare workers are easily among the most stressful of any industry. Consider the stressors:
- The core activity is helping patients who may or may not be able to have a "good outcome."
- Healthcare workers interact with people—either patients or family members—often facing the most emotional times/events of their lives.
- Working with limited resources amid ever growing volumes and need for care services.
- Rapid and ever-changing industry with requirements for constant training.[104]

These factors lead to a high rate of burnout. A survey of 3,896 Mayo Clinic physicians found that 40 percent reported at least one symptom of burnout, and that burnout rates were higher in physicians who rated their leaders unfavorably. They also found that, even in a physician group with high satisfaction ratings (79 percent satisfied or very satisfied), leadership quality explained almost half the variation in physician satisfaction scores. This study highlights the importance of organizational leadership to clinician well-being. While this study reported on physician burnout, similar findings have been reported across the healthcare workforce with worrisome correlations between poor staff well-being and patient safety.[105] A *Health Affairs* study comparing patient-satisfaction scores with HCAHPS surveys of almost 100,000 nurses showed that a better nurse work environment was associated with higher scores on every patient-satisfaction survey question. And University of Pennsylvania professor Linda Aiken found that higher staffing of registered nurses has been linked to fewer patient deaths and improved quality of health. Failure-to-rescue rates drop. Patients are less likely to die or to get readmitted to the hospital. Their hospital stay is shorter and their likelihood of being the victim of a fatigue-related error is lower. When hospitals improve nurse working conditions, rather than tricking patients into believing they're getting better care, the quality of care really does get better.[106]

In addition to lower quality care, staff burnout indicates a staff that is likely to turn-over and increases the challenge in cultivating a culture of compassion to deliver care that is *Heartwired*. For registered nurses the chance of compassion fatigue and burnout continues to rise. According to the *2016 National Healthcare Retention & RN Staffing Report* turnover for bedside RNs in 2014 was 16.4 percent, and rose to 17.2 percent in 2015.[107] Certified nursing assistants recorded the highest rate at 23.8 percent. Constant replacement and retraining of staff to achieve high-quality work performance is expensive and time consuming. Creating a *Heartwired* culture of support will increase chances of improving outcomes for healthcare workers leading to improved outcomes for patients and families. Much like the care we want them to deliver, we need to be five stars in our support of healthcare workers.

Heartwiring is not an acronym to be memorized, or a one-off system-wide campaign. Rather, *Heartwiring* should become the inbred culture of compassion among your healthcare providers and all who work across the healthcare system. Successful teams will need time to work together as they develop a culture of compassion with low rates of burnout. Once achieved, they will need sufficient time to support the culture and reinforce it by introducing it to new associates who are the next to become *Heartwired*. The Toolkit that follows this chapter has resources for developing a *Heartwired* culture.

As we learned in Chapter 7, when Dr. Bridget Duffy took the helm as Chief Experience Officer at The Cleveland Clinic, she told leaders they had to be willing to address the underlying culture of the organization. She was asking them to allow her to fix more than the low HCAHPS scores. She knew they were symptomatic of more than simple performances mistakes. Her answer might have surprised many, but given all we've learned so far, it makes sense. Dr Duffy felt the answer was to "restore joy" to the practice of medicine and to do that she proposed to move beyond the IHI's Triple Aim and aspire to a Quadruple Aim.

FOR BETTER OUTCOMES, ADD ONE PART JOY

Dr. Duffy's recommendation to "restore joy" might sound more applicable to the Magic Kingdom than a healthcare system, but for healthcare workers on the verge of burnout, it is just what the doctor ordered. The Experience Innovation Network (EIN), an international group of Chief Experience Officers (CXOs) and other health system executives focused on patient and care team experience, is dedicated to helping providers meet what we call the "Quadruple Aim," using human-centered design principles to identify technologies that optimize the patient-physician encounter, which will help restore joy back to the practice of medicine. The Quadruple Aim builds on IHI's Triple Aim—improving patient experience, improving population health, and decreasing the cost of care—by adding a fourth measure focused on achieving joy, well-being, and resilience among care teams, including physicians.

To this end, the US should appoint a Chief Experience Officer (CXO)—on par with the Surgeon General—to oversee efforts to re-center the person as the primary focus of healthcare. This will include:

- Restoring empathy, efficiency, and quality to healthcare;
- Promoting human-centered design principles with patients as partners;
- Deploying technologies that build trust and ease the burden of being a clinician;
- Embedding patients as "Experience Co-Design Fellows" in all hospitals and clinics nationwide (replacing the underutilized patient and family advisory councils that often simply rubber stamp design plans);
- Mandating training on improving organizational culture and communication practices to ensure seamless care transitions as well as competence and compassion at every patient encounter; and
- Creating "Metrics for Humanity" that assess resiliency, joy, and well-being of care teams, and are applied to technologies that improve the outcome and experience of both staff and patients.

With sufficient legislative and programmatic infrastructure, these activities would help us transform our fragmented healthcare system beyond the "Triple Aim" of improving patient experience and health while reducing per capita healthcare costs. We can and should pursue the "Quadruple

Aim" that includes restoring joy back to the practice of medicine, using a truly interdisciplinary approach that addresses the inherent trauma of the system and liberates people from bureaucracy. Key to that approach is a thoughtful examination of how the right types of process improvement and technology—leveraged in the right ways—can counter burnout rates while also improving the healthcare experience for both care teams and patients.[108]

So how can we move to having more *Heartwired* associates and fewer burned out associates? Like they say, it all starts with acknowledging there's a problem. Bring the reality of burnout into the light and let your clinicians know you want to be part of their support system as well. Acknowledge compassion fatigue and the need for education, support, and even respite among your professional providers. Some strategies are discussed below.

Share the "Story of the Stone Masons" and discuss its three important strategies to *Heartwired* success:

1. **Start with Your Why**
   What is the shared purpose of your organization? This leads to hiring decisions and training strategies that support a shared culture of excellence. This unified strategy aligns leadership and associates together toward desired outcomes. Find those bricklayers who believe they are building your cathedral!

2. **Attitude is Everything!**
   Is your glass half full or half empty?
   Each of us is in complete control of one thing each and every day: We can choose an attitude of compassion and positivity and contribute to the best outcomes possible for our patients and families. Or, we can go another way.

3. **See the Big Picture: It's a Cathedral!**
   One brick, two bricks, three bricks; No wall gets made without a brick. No cathedral gets made without a wall. Being able to see the end result, and knowing how your task contributes, provides motivation to excel. For the Medical Assistant rooming a patient

on time helps keep the clinic running on time and leads to a five-star experience. At times our focus is only on the immediate task. When we change our focus to the bigger picture, this perspective provides motivation to continue as well as to continually improve performance for the sake of the patient, the outcome, and the team.

CONVENE SCHWARTZ ROUNDS

In Chapter 9, we quoted the remarkable Mr. Kenneth Schwartz, the late author of *A Patient's Story* published by The Boston Globe in 1991. Through his story he gave voice to the experience of being a patient and exposed the need for increased compassion in healthcare. Sadly, he figured this out after being given less-than-compassionate care at times. He was a keen observer paying attention as he moved through various healthcare settings. He saw how hard it is for professional caregivers to be compassionate while under time pressures. He saw how poor communication can frustrate both caregivers and patients alike, fracturing relationships, disengaging caregivers, and leading to suboptimal care. Fortunately for all of us, while Ken Schwartz was seeing these problems, he was also envisioning a solution.

> At the end of his life, Ken outlined the organization he wanted to create. It would be a center that would nurture compassion in healthcare, encouraging the sorts of caregiver-patient relationships that made all the difference to him. He founded the Schwartz Center in 1995–just days before his death–to ensure that all patients receive compassionate and humane care.
>
> The Schwartz Center for Compassionate Healthcare's mission is simple but compelling: to promote compassionate care so that patients and their caregivers relate to one another in a way that provides hope to the patient, support to caregivers and sustenance to the healing process.[109]

Today the Schwartz Center serves as an important leader in promoting increased compassion across healthcare. An excerpt from their website:

Supporting Providers. Improving Quality of Care
The stresses of today's healthcare system threaten the delivery of compassionate care. Financial pressures and administrative demands mean less time with patients and a focus on diagnosis and treatment rather than the impact an illness can have on the patient and family. Many caregivers today are anxious, frustrated and under pressure—with no structured outlet for expressing their feelings and little preparation for the difficult communication issues that are an inevitable part of patient care.

The Schwartz Rounds® program, now taking place in more than 470 healthcare organizations throughout the US, Canada, Australia, New Zealand, and more than 190 sites throughout the UK and Ireland, offers healthcare providers a regularly scheduled time during their fast-paced work lives to openly and honestly discuss the social and emotional issues they face in caring for patients and families. In contrast to traditional medical rounds, the focus is on the human dimension of medicine. Caregivers have an opportunity to share their experiences, thoughts and feelings on thought-provoking topics drawn from actual patient cases. The premise is that caregivers are better able to make personal connections with patients and colleagues when they have greater insight into their own responses and feelings.

A hallmark of the program is interdisciplinary dialogue. Panelists from diverse disciplines participate in the sessions, including physicians, nurses, social workers, psychologists, allied health professionals and chaplains. After listening to a panel's brief presentation on an identified case or topic, caregivers in the audience are invited to share their own perspectives on the case and broader related issues.

In order to conduct Schwartz Rounds, your healthcare institution must be a healthcare member of the Schwartz Center for Compassionate Healthcare. Membership information can be found on their website:

https://www.theschwartzcenter.org/programs/schwartz-rounds

DO YOU HAVE SOLAR PANELS OR GAS TANKS?

In his superb lecture series, *Mind-Body Medicine: The New Science of Optimal Health*, Professor Satterfield relays the story of a medical school professor who annually greeted incoming medical students with their first lesson in "perspective shifting" for young medical students entering the stressful workplace of modern healthcare. The seasoned physician describes how he shifts his mindset as he enters a room or begins a provider-patient encounter.

> Let's assume you are a busy internist and you go to see your first patient and you have a gas tank [...] you roll up your sleeves, you get to work, it's a complicated case, but you figure it out... You prescribe the right medication and burn off a little fuel, you go to the next patient, work and work really hard, make a tough diagnosis and burn off more fuel, move to the next patient, and again work really hard, burn off more fuel, go to the next patient. And by the end of the day your tank is on empty and you are exhausted and you go home to your family exhausted.
>
> Your partner, Physician #2, has a solar panel. This physician is also a busy internist in the same practice. He goes to see his first patient...it is a complicated case and there is a lot of work to do, but in that moment they have the presence of mind to remember that they are in a privileged position, that they are doing something that matters, that they have a skillset that is going to affect another person, that their interventions, their decisions, their collaborations might make a difference in someone else's

life […] in that moment that privilege radiates on their solar panels and they feel charged! They go to see the next patient; they are present and they feel that connection. They go to see the next patient and they again feel that connection with another human being […] at the end of their day they are physically tired, but their soul is full and that is what they take home to their family.

Which type of physician are you? Which type would you like to be? How about the people you work with and lead? Leaders can help each associate think about whether they are a gas tank employee or solar panel employee. *Heartwired* employees will have the solar panels.

KEEP A GRATITUDE JOURNAL

A strategy to combat work stress is to replace it with positive emotion. An exercise Dr. Satterfield discusses is a good example of how to do this:

> A group of medical students was asked to participate in a study evaluating stress levels and the impact of keeping what was called a "Gratitude Journal." Students were asked to journal daily by answering these 3 questions: What surprised you today? What moved you? What inspired you? From this simple daily act, students experienced decreased stress.

The opportunity to achieve a core culture change is embedded deep within these recommendations and will help you *Heartwire* associates for a lasting change.

CONCLUSION

Putting it All together—*Heartwiring* for Healthcare Excellence
Have you ever worked very hard alongside other people and absolutely loved every minute of it, even though you were physically exhausted at the end of the day? If so, what made it so enjoyable? When asked this question, Fred would talk about the time when his family spent its traditional week at his wife's mother's house in Medford, Oregon.

When Fred's mother-in-law was in her 80s, she lived alone on a small social security check. Her three daughters and their families would descend sometime in the spring and spend strenuous days planting a huge garden to give grandma another year of produce. They would paint what needed painting. They repaired things that were broken. One time, the roof needed new shingles. Another time, grab rails were installed where she had precarious footing. Later a front porch banister was installed as she became less steady on her feet. In addition to the repairs completed, what they all remembered was the joy, the utter happiness they felt in hard work. Nobody needed a boss. Family members of all ages pitched in where extra hands were needed. Someone went to the market. Someone cooked wonderful, wholesome meals, made more delicious by hearty appetites.

Children found plenty to do and cheerfully joined in. They weeded the flowerbeds and washed windows and scrubbed floors without being bribed or coerced to do so. In fact, offering money would have diminished their intrinsic motivation—the fun of working with loved ones—that fueled all the efforts and brought pleasure in the hard work that made it possible for grandma to continue living in her little house on Peach Street. Ultimately she was able to live there until she was 91 years old, when a fall required her to sell her home and live with one of her daughters.

If asked to describe the perfect work environment, what factors would you include?

1. Doing something important for someone else who cannot do it for themselves?
2. Having an unsurpassed level of joy in hard work with good people?

What comes closer to this picture than being a caregiver in a hospital? The question is, how does one create such a team, and maintain such a spirit?

DREAMS MOTIVATE

For many old enough to have witnessed it, a program broadcast across the country on August 28, 1963, became a lifelong memory. For many, the event led them to act. Though they didn't have the benefit of social media to attract a crowd, on that day Martin Luther King, Jr. stood on the steps of the Lincoln Memorial in Washington, DC, and spoke to the 200,000 people amassed around him. He gave what is now regarded as one of the greatest speeches of all time. It has become known as the famous, "I Have a Dream" speech. Millions of Americans from all walks of life were stirred as they listened to a descendant of slaves say, "I have a dream that one day this nation will rise up and live out the true meaning of its creed: 'We hold these truths to be self-evident: that all men are created equal'… I have a dream that my four little children will one day live in a nation where they will not be judged by the color of their skin but by the content of their character." The words still echo and have inspired many since that pivotal day.

Notably, Martin Luther King, Jr. did not say, "I have a strategic initiative." He did not say, "I have a business plan." Somehow, we know it would not have been very inspiring if he had. Plans and initiatives, and most mission statements, do not inspire people. It is articulating a dream that inspires commitment and motivation. Carl Sandburg wrote, "Nothing happens unless first a dream." Certainly, Walt Disney was primarily a dreamer of great dreams. Armed with those dreams, he inspired talented people to share his dreams and make them a reality. When people are part of a team that is inspired by the same dream, they will do their own initiating and planning.

Start with your own dream by remembering a time when you loved working with other people. Analyze what made the experience so great. Then translate those principles into your current work environment by sharing that dream with your team every day. Encourage your team to create its own dream. We spend time crafting our strategic plans each year, so next time do a little dreaming first

IF YOU CAN DREAM IT

Ask a series of behavioral statements that indicate the elements that must come together to create the dream. It might look like this:

I dream of working in a department where:
- We all feel like friends you can trust;
- We find meaning in our work;
- As a team we have a shared vision;
- We create the best experience for our patients (or customers);
- We contribute to the overall success of our organization.

Next, present these statements to the people who report to you and have them share their thoughts. Create your team's dream. Later by taking each of the five statements separately, you have a springboard for important conversations about what it would take to make that statement a reality.

For instance, the statement that says, "We create the best experience for our patients (or customers)," ask each team member in the group to complete the following statements:

I can best help the team by _____.
I need support from the team for _____.

You may also want to ask each individual to privately complete:

I enjoy my work when the team _____.

I wish there was less _____.
I wish there was more _____.

This process of collectively probing for information and having frank conversations can be the foundation for improved teamwork and achievement.

CHOOSE THE RIGHT WORDS WITH THE RIGHT MEANINGS

Words are more than representations of thoughts. They actually shape our thoughts. Here are some words that have shaped our collective thoughts about leadership for many years. Yet each of them gives us a connotation that falls short if we want a *Heartwired* culture. We've added a "*Heartwired*" term you can start using to help shape you or your team's thoughts in that direction.

The Old Term → The *Heartwired* Term

Service → Experience
We are not at a patient's bedside to provide a service. We are there to provide a compassionate healing experience so the body can mend itself.

Leadership → Culture
Leadership still implies a "leader" from whom most or all direction flows. Culture implies a shared vision leading our words, actions, and decisions.

Empowerment → Ownership
We need employees who take ownership of the values that define a committed work culture in the same way that we need citizens who take ownership of the values of society.

Accountability → Responsibility
Citizens who take ownership will act responsibly. They give up some of their own freedom in order to take responsibility for the success of the whole.

Starts at the top → Starts anywhere and everywhere
We need to get rid of the notion that it must "start at the top." The truth is, it can start anywhere. Folks at "the top" need to encourage and support a culture of citizens who take ownership and responsibility because, ideally, all associates *Heartwired* to care with compassion will create the ways in which the corporate culture lives out its dream of creating an unforgettable experience for patients and caregivers.

EXCELLENCE IS FUN

Anything done at the level of excellence, or in the pursuit of excellence, is exciting and fun. Anything done at the level of mediocrity is discouraging and a real drag. Where there is low morale, we often make low pay or hard work the scapegoats. More often it is a combination of factors, perhaps the dispiriting effect of poor team performance, silent competition between silos, the disengagement of under-resourced departments, finger-pointing negativity, and/or uninspired leadership. The best way to break this vicious cycle is for leadership to support the culture of *Heartwired* excellence with their own efforts starting with why and moving forward with continuous quality improvement toward ever greater performance. Set the standard, provide the resources, hold all accountable to processes and outcomes, and then ask associates to follow suit. Challenge them to become better and better in an area they all believe is important and supports your collective goals.

Nothing inspires like success. There is nothing like becoming excellent at something to meet our basic drive for competence and feed our deep hunger for meaning and growth. This is the source of passion. Knowing and believing this truth about human motivation can make an ordinary manager a great coach. Start with a dream then lead toward excellence. The continuous quality improvement cycles are good opportunities to allow teams to take action. As we learned earlier, taking action, even if it is not the final version of how your team might operate, allows improvement if you are actively engaged in the PDSA cycle.

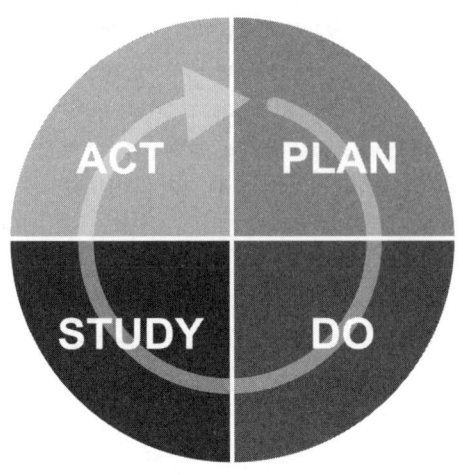

Heartwiring Healthcare Excellence

Plan	Define Excellence
Do	Do Something to Improve
Study	Check the Results
Act	Analyze it, and Do it again, and again

Improving our ability to learn from our mistakes actually improves our skills of analysis and decision-making skills, which will often make us better at the very thing we "failed" at. All of this fuels the excitement and fun on the way toward performance excellence. There would be no science, no technology, no discipline, no product of any kind, were it not for someone who worked diligently to learn from their failures, find solutions, and share the success.

Leaders can make it happen for a healthcare system. Managers can make it happen for their work unit. Individuals can make it happen for themselves. Collectively, we can create healthcare systems *Heartwired* for Healthcare Excellence.

HEARTWIRING TOOLKIT

"All our dreams can come true if we have the courage to pursue them."
~ Walt Disney

Heartwired healthcare. Sounds good, doesn't it? It's the type of care we all would want for our loved ones. It's how we'd want to be treated when it's our turn to be the patient. And a **Heartwired hospital** is just the type of place we would all like to work.

Creating a *Heartwired* culture where compassion and empathy are the default should be "job one" for all of us in healthcare. And "job two"? Sustaining it!

It will take many of us working together toward the dream of *Heartwired* healthcare. We can each be leaders of this important movement. First, we can lead ourselves to be *Heartwired*. We can be a model for others and help the compassion contagion spread! Those in leadership roles can provide critically important vision and mission, organizational infrastructure, and frontline support for developing and sustaining a *Heartwired* culture.

In this Toolkit we provide tactics to support change on both an individual and system level. We encourage you to find the mix that best fits your setting and needs. Before looking at the specific strategies let's talk about one of the most vexing aspects of organizational performance. Change.

After all, for most of us to become fully *Heartwired* will require some changes. For most of our healthcare systems to become fully *Heartwired* will require changes. Deciding you want to be *Heartwired* and work in a *Heartwired* healthcare system is the first step. As you plan to disseminate and work toward change, we recommend you review a key tenet of change management, accountability.

Successful change requires:
1. A focused and clearly stated goal to be achieved from the change; Consider setting so-called "SMART" goals.

SMART goal; **S**pecific, **M**easurable, **A**ttainable, **R**elevant, **T**imely[110]

The *SMART* acronym first appeared in the November 1981 issue of Management Review, "There's a *S.M.A.R.T.* way to write management *goals* and *objectives*," was the article's title and it was written by George Doran, Arthur Miller, and James Cunningham.

2. Leadership and associate dedication to spend the time and resources required to meet the goal;
3. Accountability of all toward doing the work required to change AND achieving the goal.

Each of us must keep focused on the goal of becoming *Heartwired*; dedicate ourselves to spending time and resources in support of the goal, and holding our work teams and ourselves accountable. This approach will make all the difference between your efforts for system improvements being seen as the "flavor-of-the month" and making lasting change for good.

Done correctly, *Heartwiring* can reframe healthcare as a profession imbued with compassion and empathy. So how can we lead successful change and hold each other accountable as we embark on *Heartwiring* our systems and ourselves? Let's first look outside healthcare at some valuable advice about changing human thought and behavior.

Hitting the news in 2018 and 2019 were some highly publicized events exposing continuing societal biases about race. Well-known companies including Starbucks and Sephora have "shut-down" the company to hold all-hands-on-deck programs to try and address these shortcomings active within their corporate culture and operations. Likely there was some value in these programs, but unfortunately most failed to create lasting and sustained change. In 2017 the Harvard Business Review article of the year was "Why Diversity Programs Fail," by sociology professors Frank Dobbin and Alexandra Kalev.

https://www.mckinsey.com/about-us/new-at-mckinsey-blog/mckinsey-award-winners-why-diversity-programs-fail-and-what-world-war-ii-can-teach-us-about-success

The key message is the need to go beyond raising awareness to creating an ongoing effort aimed at continuing desired skills, attitudes, and behaviors. Dr. Kalev summarizes:

> What works better is a diversity committee or task force, made up of people from the organization from different departments and different ranks. They come together, examine their own department or function or team, and learn of specific barriers to diversity. Then they develop tailored solutions, follow the implementation, and, ideally, report on progress. It's a sustained effort."

Dobbins and Kalev's work shows the power of focusing effort across the organization from top leadership to frontline associates. The best path toward sustained success uses this integrated group to focus change efforts with ongoing disciplined review and revision. Implicit in Dobbins and Kaley's recommendations is the need for top leadership to endorse the need for and value of the cultural change. In his seminal work on change management, Harvard's John Kotter used the phrase "leading change" as he described the 8-step process of the endeavor. Anchored by a leadership vision and urgency, the 8 steps create a foundation for progress that can produce effective and sustained change.

KOTTER'S 8-STEP PROCESS

https://www.kotterinc.com/8-steps-process-for-leading-change/

Create a sense of urgency
Build a guiding coalition
Form a strategic vision and initiatives
Enlist a volunteer army
Enable action by removing barriers
Generate short-term wins
Sustain acceleration
Institute change

For a healthcare system to become *Heartwired*, leaders and associates need to step forward and promote compassion and empathy as an expected attribute of all they do. Where compassion and empathy are valued and expected, it will become the norm. As *Heartwired* leaders and associates hold each other accountable, change will be sustained. The collective power of individual associates will allow a *Heartwired* culture to thrive as each *Heartwired* associate acts as a force multiplier providing *Heartwired* care AND inspiring fellow associates to become *Heartwired* too!

Finally, back in Chapter 2 we learned about strategies for continuous quality improvement from W. Edwards Deming. The powerful PDSA cycle encourages us to constantly evaluate how we operate and provide care using the Plan, Do, Study, and Act cycles to move us toward sustainable success. We believe this is make or break on the road to becoming and staying *Heartwired*. Review PDSA if need be and use the concept regularly. Across a healthcare system, small work groups can work to ensure *Heartwired* healthcare thrives.

HINTS FOR *HEARTWIRING*:
Compassion + Empathy = *Heartwired*

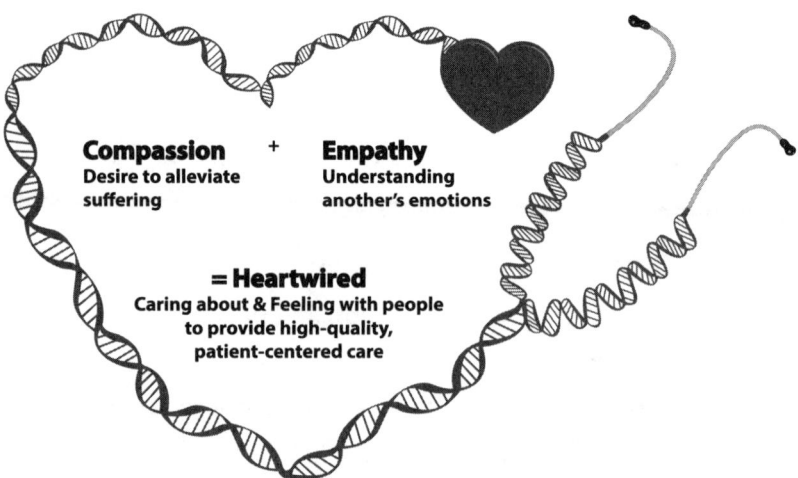

Compassion
Desire to alleviate suffering

+

Empathy
Understanding another's emotions

= Heartwired
Caring about & Feeling with people to provide high-quality, patient-centered care

Creating any workplace culture depends on creating a shared/collective set of beliefs, standards of behavior, and mutual expectations. Perhaps when we think about changing something as large, dynamic, and complex as a healthcare system, we first think about leaders from a central authority taking responsibility for setting and disseminating cultural standards among their frontline staff. That will not do here. *Heartwiring* is not a top-down phenomenon. It is an innately personal expression of compassion and empathy. The power of *Heartwiring* lies in the potential energy of the person displaying that compassion and empathy. Just one person can influence another who will influence another and so on, until ultimately there is a *Heartwired* culture across the healthcare system. Beyond their ability to influence fellow associates, there are other benefits to increasing the ranks of *Heartwired* associates.

Heartwired associates will be:
- Resilient and able to adapt to stressors
- Sources of compassion and empathy for patients
- Role models for fellow associates

Throughout the book we described ways each of us can individually supplement our natural compassion and fortify ourselves as we move within the stressful environments and challenging interpersonal interactions of healthcare. Let's review some of the key lessons we can use for ourselves or those we want to lead toward being *Heartwired*. As more of us choose to be *Heartwired*, we will inspire and lead others to do the same.

INSPIRING INDIVIDUALS

"I alone cannot change the world, but I can cast a stone across the waters to create many ripples."
~ Mother Teresa

What does it take to motivate you to make a change? Certainly, we all need to be convinced there is value in making the change. Otherwise why go to all that effort? Making change on an individual level requires making a connection to a core value and an outcome that we hold in high regard. Included below are some of the best strategies we've come across. Consider using these to motivate key associates across the healthcare system. Once they shift toward being *Heartwired*, they will act as change agents and efforts will multiply.

Do you have Solar panels or a Gas Tank? *Chapter 10, page 139*
In his superb lecture series *Mind-Body Medicine: The New Science of Optimal Health*, Professor Jason Satterfield relays the story of a medical school professor who annually greeted incoming medical students entering the stressful workplace of modern healthcare with their first lesson in "perspective shifting". The seasoned (and masterly, in our minds) physician **describes how he shifts his mindset—to one that is more *Heartwired*—as he enters a room or begins a provider-patient encounter.**

> Let's assume you are a busy internist and you go to see your first patient and you have a gas tank. You roll up your sleeves, you get to work, it's a complicated case but you figure it out. You prescribe the right medication and burn off a little fuel. You go to the next patient, work and work really hard, make a tough diagnosis and burn off more fuel, move to the next patient, and again work really hard, burn off more fuel, go to the next patient. And by the end of the day your tank is on empty and you are exhausted, and you go home to your family exhausted.
>
> Your partner, Physician #2, has a solar panel. This physician is also a busy internist in the same practice. He goes to see his first patient. It is a complicated case and there is a lot of work to do, but in that moment they have the presence of mind to remember that they are in a privileged position that they are doing something that matters. They have a skillset that is going to affect another person, they know that their interventions, their decisions, their collaborations might make a difference in someone else's life. In that moment, that privilege radiates on their solar panels and they feel charged! They go to see the next patient; they are present, and they feel that connection. They go to see the next patient and they again feel that connection with another

human being. At the end of their day they are physically tired, but their soul is full and that is what they take home to their family.

Which type of associate are you? Do you have solar panels or gas tanks? Which type would you like to be? How about the people you work with and lead? *Heartwired* employees will have the solar panels.

THE STARFISH STORY AND THE POWER OF ONE

Heartwired associates will have influence in several important ways. First, they will help those they are personally caring for. As we learned in Chapter 6 (Take Two Placebos and Call Me in the Morning), the one-to-one human interactions of healthcare are themselves vitally important to the overall healing process. Next, the associates will serve as role models for valuing that individual benefit. The University of Pennsylvania academic and renowned essayist, Loren Eiseley, PhD, is credited with authoring the parable of the starfish to describe the awesome power existing in but one human being whose actions can have vast and multiple influences.

> An old man had a habit of early morning walks on the beach. One day, after a storm, he saw a human figure in the distance moving like a dancer. As he came closer, he saw that it was a young woman and she was not dancing but was reaching down to the sand, picking up a starfish and very gently throwing them into the ocean. "Young lady," he asked, "Why are you throwing starfish into the ocean?" "The sun is up, and the tide is going out, and if I do not throw them in, they will die." "But young lady, do you not realize that there are miles and miles of beach and starfish all along it? You cannot possibly make a difference." The young woman listened politely, paused and then bent down, picked up another starfish and threw it into the sea, past the breaking waves, saying, "It made a difference for that one." The old man looked at the young woman inquisitively and thought

about what she had done. Inspired, he joined her in throwing starfish back into the sea. Soon others joined, and all the starfish were saved.[111]

The young lady is *Heartwired*. And by saving the starfish she has shown the old man the power of one to influence. First her influence saved individual starfish, but soon her influence saved many through her influence of others. That is how one *Heartwired* associate will influence a healthcare system one patient at a time. Soon the system will have many patients being treated by *Heartwired* associates.

PAY IT FORWARD—*Chapter 7, pages 93-94*

Altruism is a powerful thing. Our human psyche gets a real charge when we are altruistic. And anyone observing the altruistic act will be inspired to do the same. It's that good. In Chapter 7 we learned just how this valuable trait was created in an evolutionary sense. Back in the days of the sabertooth tiger, compassion among humans set the stage for survival. Helping each other and relying on the kindness of others helped people stay alive. Our brain recognizes suffering and unfairness and triggers the "caretaking" center—the vagus nerve—that stimulates a range of actions across the body from our brain to heart and lungs that diminish distressing symptoms. So, some of this compassion comes naturally and those who display it play a key role in inspiring others with their compassion. In her book *Pay it Forward*, author Catherine Rand Hyde introduced the concept of acting kindly at the individual level serving a dual purpose of helping the individual and motivating others to do the same thus creating more kindness. This kind of grass-roots effort can be a powerful movement across a healthcare system where opportunities to help a patient or fellow associate are plentiful. As the altruism spreads you will be well on your way to create a *Heartwired* culture across the system.

"Pay it Forward—The Healthcare Edition" is a quick way to inspire one person or many to practice random acts of kindness as a step toward *Heartwiring* the system. Quick! Pick a number between one and fifteen:

Got it? Now find that Pay it Forward idea below and do it.

1. Pay it Backward: offer to pay for the person behind you in the cafeteria line.
2. Compliment the first three people you talk to today.
3. Post inspirational sticky notes around the unit, your break room, a patient's room, etc.
4. Surprise co-workers with freshly baked cookies or a favorite treat.
5. Encounter someone who is especially kind? Take an extra five minutes to tell their manager.
6. Smile at five strangers.
7. Set an alarm on your phone to go off at three different times during the day. In those moments, do something kind for someone else.
8. Send a gratitude e-mail to a coworker who deserves more recognition. Copy their boss.
9. Practice self-kindness and spend thirty minutes doing something you love today.
10. Write a gratitude list in the morning and again in the evening.
11. Everyone is important. Learn the names of your office security guard, the person at the front desk, and other people you see every day. Greet them by name. Also say "hello" to strangers and smile. These acts of kindness are so easy, and they almost always make people smile.
12. Find opportunities to give compliments. It costs nothing, takes no time, and could make someone's entire day. Don't just think it. Say it.
13. Ask a busy coworker if you can do something to help.
14. Put your phone away while in the company of others.
15. When you hear that discouraging voice in your head, tell yourself something positive—you deserve kindness too!

(adapted from the Random Acts of Kindness Foundation's blog post https://www.randomactsofkindness.org/the-kindness-blog/2917-50-ways-to-pay-it-forward)

INSPIRING TEAMS OF ASSOCIATES

"Never doubt that a small group of thoughtful committed citizens can change the world; indeed, it's the only thing that ever has."
~ Margaret Mead

What does it take to motivate a group of people to change? What the celebrated American cultural anthropologist Margaret Mead identified was the fact that cooperation is among our defining characteristics as a species. Back in the hunter-gatherer days a loner would not survive, but teams working the hunt would obtain sufficient food. In his article *Working Together is Part of What Makes us Human*,[112] Dr. John Parrington presents evidence that as a species, humans are far more inclined to cooperation than competition, the need to comfort the sick and help the disabled comes naturally. Our proto-human ancestors were already caring for the long-term sick and disabled people! So, if it's human nature to behave with compassion and empathy why do we have to teach people to do it? And why would we have to teach people how to show it? Because in our modern healthcare systems caring often occurs in time-crunched and complex settings demanding attention to the clock as much as attention to the patient. Providing compassion and empathy in this situation requires new skills. *Heartwired* associates have those skills and can be highly successful mentors for others. Key *Heartwired* associates can lead small work teams focused on *Heartwiring* the care they provide. Once several teams start the journey others will see their outcomes and experiences and want to join in. Let's look at ways to harness the cooperative spirit of individuals to create highly compassionate, empathetic, and *Heartwired* teams.

We recommend a "retreat" model with learners **completely** apart from usual responsibilities as well as digital or mobile distractions. Set yourself up for success by ensuring all involved can be fully present and engaged. That lesson alone will be a step toward a *Heartwired* culture. Be purposeful in letting associates know what the purpose of the "retreat" is. While the most common definition of retreat is to back away from a fight, that's definitely not what we are doing here! Quite the opposite, really. Retreats are also periods of time for careful thought and a change from previous beliefs or behavior. In the quest for *Heartwired* healthcare a retreat can be an ideal setting for full discussion of this challenging topic, introducing new perspectives and developing skills to foster and sustain a *Heartwired* culture across the healthcare system.

Here we provide some templates and content you may find useful for retreat planning.

Sample 3-hour Retreat: *Heartwiring* **Healthcare**
Introduces the general concepts and begins individual and team-based skills development.

Hour 1	Compassionate Caring
Hour 2	The Basis of Empathy
Hour 3	*Heartwired* for Good

Sample 6-hour Retreat: Heartwiring _____ (Insert Your Hospital Name Here)
Extends the concept and work of Heartwiring to your specific institution.

Hours	1-3 from above
Hour 4	Compassion is Contagious
Hour 5	We Walk in Your Shoes
Hour 6	*Heartwired* Forever

Content Samples for 3-hour retreat "*Heartwiring* Healthcare"
Program notes: Each "hour" will have fifty minutes of content followed by ten minutes to transition to next topic.

Hour 1: Compassionate Caring
Introduction
Welcome and Ground Rules
- Confidentiality
- Listening without judgment
- Everyone is "off the grid"; No one in the room is "on call"

The basic goal of *Heartwiring* Healthcare is to allow compassion and empathy to emerge as the leading forces creating fully therapeutic relationships that heal and nurture our patients. We will work together to learn skills to provide compassionate and empathetic care each and every time, and no matter how complicated, time-pressured, and chaotic events around us are. We will be *Heartwired*!

Exercise: Mini Schwartz Rounds—45 minutes

In Chapter 9 we introduced you to the prescient and altruistic Mr. Ken Schwartz who, as he was dying, wanted to do what he could to ensure others had compassionate care during their time of need. His belief was that the strengthening of the human connection was at the heart of compassionate healthcare. Following his death, Schwartz Rounds have become a leading program offering of the Schwartz Center for Compassionate Healthcare. Practiced now across the globe, Schwartz Rounds create a foundation for human connection with compassion. In this exercise, you can introduce attendees to the philosophy of Schwartz Rounds and then give them an opportunity to participate in one.

Watch this video (7:42 minutes):

https://www.theschwartzcenter.org/supporting-caregivers/schwartz-center-rounds/

Topic Introduction: Mini Schwartz Rounds

Choose from among the attendees to create a panel of three different disciplines (if possible) and ask each person to take three minutes to answer these prompts:
- Describe a patient you feel you made an especially strong connection of caring with.
- What made the difference for that relationship? Were there any challenges to making the connection?
- Encourage input and reflection from the audience focusing on strategies to create and foster healing relationships.

- Give each panelist a maximum of three minutes to share their experience and then allow a maximum of ten minutes of group reflection = 3 x 13 minutes total = 39 min (+ 7:42 to watch video above) = about 47 minutes total

Hour 2: The Basis of Empathy
Introduction (ten minutes)
The Daisy Story
Materials:
- White board and pen
- Daisy—Silk Shasta daisy stems available at craft stores.
- Three Power point slides: full Shasta daisy, next with petals falling, last with bare stem

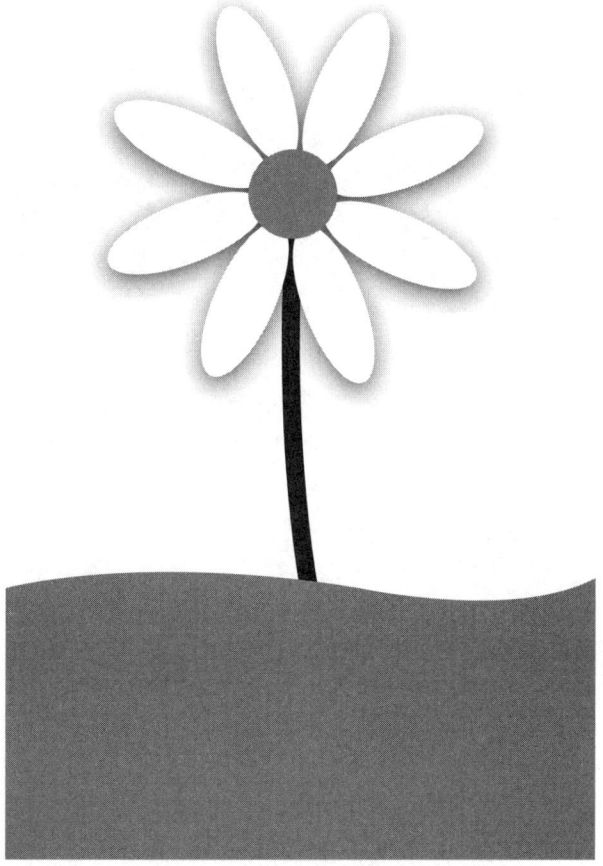

Instructions: As described in Chapter 5
- Encourage all attendees to hold the flower and think about all of their life's blessings
- Ask the group to share and write the main categories on the white board

Lessons Learned:
- We cannot imagine what we don't truly know.
- We will likely underestimate the challenges of others.
- We need to respect the fact that most of our patients have suffered beyond what we know or have experience with ourselves.

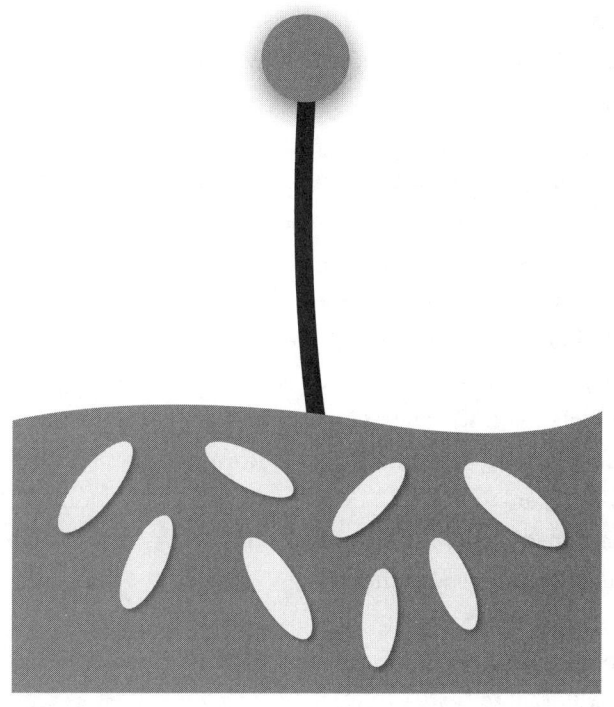

Exercise: 35 minutes.

Watch the Cleveland Clinic commercial (4:24 minutes)
https://www.google.com/search?q=cleveland+clinic+empathy+commercial&oq=cleveland+clinic+empathy+commercial&aqs=chrome..69i57.9494j1j7&sourceid=chrome&ie=UTF-8

Discussion questions—ten minutes per question
1. Which person's caption surprised you the most?
2. Which patient can you relate to?
3. What can we do differently in day-to-day care to keep in mind the "walk in their shoes" perspective?

Hour 3 Heartwiring for Good?

Introduction: The Clock Story—five minutes

There was a small town that had all the usual institutions. It had a bathhouse, cemetery, hospital, and a court of law as well as all sorts of craftsmen. It had tailors, dressmakers, carpenters, masons and so on. One trade however was lacking, there was no watchmaker.

Now as the years went by many of the clocks became so inaccurate that their owners just decided to let them run down and ignored them altogether. There were others, however, who maintained that as long as their clock ran, they should not be abandoned. So, they wound their clocks day after day even though they knew they were not accurate. One day news spread through the town that a watchmaker had arrived. Everyone rushed to him with their clocks. However, the only ones he could repair were the ones that had been kept running. The abandoned clocks were so full of rust and corrosion that he could do nothing with them.

Moral of the story: To create and sustain a *Heartwired* culture we will want to "wind the clock" day after day. We must not fail to take active steps to keep the *Heartwired* culture alive and well no matter the obstacles in the way.

Exercise: Creating a "*Heartwired* for Good" Task Force

Split the group into work teams of approximately five to seven individuals.

Explain they are to create one PDSA quality improvement project.

They will have 30 minutes to do the following:
Clarify Group Leadership
- Task Force Leader
- Facilitator

Identify Strategy
- In two to three bullet points, describe what your Task Force will do to stay "*Heartwired* for good"

SMART Goals:
- Provide two to three SMART goals

90-Day Deliverables:
- Provide two to three deliverables to accomplish in the next ninety days

Small Teamwork—30 min

Reporting—15 min

ABOUT THE AUTHORS

FRED LEE

Fred Lee was born in Kunming, China to American missionary parents, who were also born in China. Fred and his family spent many years in China and spoke fluent Mandarin.

Fred began his healthcare career at Shawnee Mission Medical Center in the Kansas City area. As vice president for marketing and development, he won several national awards for innovative approaches to patient satisfaction and loyalty. He then transitioned to be a senior vice president at Florida Hospital, one of the largest hospitals in the US, located in Orlando, Florida. There he developed a nationally acclaimed guest relations program.

Next, Disney University recruited him due to his expertise in helping hospitals achieve a culture that inspires patient and employee loyalty. He helped adapt and facilitate Disney's healthcare version of its 3-day seminar, *Disney's Approach to Quality Service*, and developed a seminar on *Customer Loyalty*.

With an insider's experience and a keen eye for cultural comparisons from his growing up in Asia and his travels around the world, Fred shared his passion and concepts of patient loyalty, the patient experience, and compassion of caregivers in his best selling book, *If Disney Ran Your Hospital: 9½ Things You Would Do Differently* which he wrote in 2004. His book was awarded the 2005 James A. Hamilton Book of the Year by the American College of Healthcare Executives. The book has become a healthcare leadership classic and has sold over 250,000 copies in English and over 250,000 books internationally, having been translated into Dutch, Portuguese, Korean, and in late 2017 into Chinese where in the last three months of 2017 became a best seller.

In 2015, Fred was appointed to the "My VA Advisory Committee" by Secretary of Veterans Affairs, Robert A. McDonald, to share his insights with US healthcare leaders.

Fred's greatest desire was for healthcare leaders and caregivers to instill his concepts for future generations. He will occupy a permanent place in American Healthcare's Pantheon of Patient Loyalty, Patient Experience, and Compassion and Empathy by caregivers.

After his first book was written in 2004 and in between his lecturing around the world, Fred spent time researching for the writing of a new book. In August of 2015 Fred was diagnosed with glioblastoma.

Fred passed away on Sunday evening, March 26, 2017.

After his passing, Fred's wife Aura and Publisher Jerry Pogue asked Dr. Laird to finish *Heartwiring*, which Fred had been working on before and during his illness. She accepted. Soon after, we began pulling all of Fred's research and worked together to bring you to the culmination of this book, *Heartwiring Healthcare Excellence*.

ROSEMARY DeANGELIS LAIRD, MD, MHSA

Dr. Laird is a Geriatrician with the AdventHealth Medical Group and is the Medical Director of the Maturing Minds Memory Disorder Clinic at AdventHealth, Orlando Florida.

She was previously the founding Medical Director of Health First Aging Services and the Center for Family Caregivers in Melbourne, Florida. Her dedication to her community, her patients, and their caregivers earned her recognition as a Space Coast Humanitarian in 2011.

Dr. Laird received her medical degree with honors from Georgetown University School of Medicine in Washington, D.C., and completed her residency in internal medicine at the University of Chicago Hospitals, where she earned the rank of Chief Resident. She then pursued a fellowship in Geriatrics at the University of Kansas, where she also earned a Masters in Health Services Administration.

A consummate advocate for seniors and family caregivers, Dr. Laird is a respected authority on the care of patients with Alzheimer's disease and other cognitive issues. She is co-author of the 2009 Best Consumer Health Book called *Take Your Oxygen First: Protecting Your Health and Happiness While Caring for a Loved One with Memory Loss*. She has authored multiple articles in peer-reviewed scientific journals. Dr. Laird is a Fellow of the American Geriatrics Society and received the Society's Clinician of the Year award in 2013. In December 2018, Dr. Laird was appointed by then Governor Rick Scott to the Florida Alzheimer's Disease Advisory Committee.

Dr. Laird began to work with Fred in his last year of life and is herself becoming known as an expert in the development of healthcare culture focused on the delivery of high-quality, compassionate, and cost-effective care, for every patient in every setting.

After Fred's passing, Fred's wife Aura, Dr. Laird, and Publisher Jerry Pogue made final plans for the book *Beyond Disney: Heartwiring Healthcare Excellence*. Dr. Laird is available for speaking appointments in the areas of developing an effective workplace culture, improving the patient experience for all patients, caring for the caregivers (both family and staff), and Alzheimer's disease.

GLOSSARY

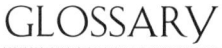

AIDET – A customer service acronym. Acknowledge the guest by name, Introduce yourself, Duration of time involved, Explain things, Thank them for choosing our hospital or clinic.

Bio-Psycho-Social – The "**bio-psycho-social model**" is an interdisciplinary model that looks at the interconnection between biology, psychology, and socio-environmental factors. The model specifically examines how these aspects play a role in topics ranging from health and disease models to human development.

CEO – Chief Executive Officer

CIO – Chief Information Officer

CMS – The Centers for Medicare and Medicaid Services

Curricula – Are the subjects of a course of study at a university or other institution.

CXO – Chief Experience Officer

Decile – Each of ten equal groups into which a population can be divided according to the distribution of values of a particular variable.

DRG – **D**iagnosis **R**elated **G**roup (**DRG**) is a patient classification system that standardizes prospective payment to hospitals. Intended to encourage cost containment, a **DRG** payment covers all charges associated with an inpatient stay from the time of admission to discharge. It is a fixed fee regardless of the actual cost incurred

Geriatrician – A geriatrician is a physician expert in the care of people 65 years of age and older. They are trained in either Family Medicine or Internal Medicine and then complete a Fellowship in Geriatrics

Glioblastoma Multiforme (GBM) Brain Tumor – **Also known as a glioblastoma**, it is a fast-growing **cancer** that develops from star-shaped glial cells (astrocytes and oligodendrocytes) that support the health of the nerve cells within the brain.

Hardwiring – An operational strategy designed to foster and ingrain the development of an organization with the culture of excellence by installing systems and processes to sustain service and operational excellence. Hardwiring was promoted in healthcare by Quint Studer in his best-selling book *Hardwiring Excellence*.

HCAHPS – The Hospital Consumer Assessment of Healthcare Providers and Systems is a patient satisfaction survey required by CMS (the Center for Medicare and Medicaid Services) for all hospitals in the United States. https://www.hcahpsonline.org/

Health Care Advisory Board – The Health Care Advisory Board is the Advisory Board's flagship research membership. It gives senior health system executives the forecasting tools and best practice insights needed to answer the industry's most pressing strategic and operational questions.

Healthcare Hall of Fame – This prestigious award is in partnership between *Modern Healthcare* magazine and the American College of Healthcare Executives (ACHE).

Institute for Healthcare Improvement (IHI) – IHI was officially founded in 1991, but its work began in the late 1980s as part of the National Demonstration Project on Quality Improvement in Health Care, led by Don Berwick, MD and a group of visionary individuals committed to redesigning healthcare into a system without errors, waste, delay, and unsustainable costs. Since then, IHI has grown from an initial collection of grant-supported programs into a self-sustaining organization with worldwide influence.

Japanese Type 2 Encephalitis – Japanese encephalitis is a neurologic infection with a broad range of manifestations. Japanese encephalitis is caused by the Japanese encephalitis virus (JEV), a flavivirus, and occurs primarily in rural areas of South and Southeast Asia. Japanese encephalitis is spread through these regions by bites of culicine mosquitoes.

Patient-Centric Healthcare – A **Patient-Centric** approach is a way in which a healthcare organization can deliver care in a tailored and personal manner that aligns with patients' wants, needs, and preferences. Where the focus is on the patient and not on the efficiency of the provider. Where care is delivered at all levels through the lens of the patient.

PDSA – **P**lan, **D**o, **S**tudy, **A**ct. See https://deming.org/uploads/paper/PDSA_History_Ron_Moen.pdf for more information.

Placebo – A placebo is an inert medical treatment or procedure able to produce a physical effect on the individual. Examples include a harmless pill, medicine, or procedure prescribed more for the psychological benefit to the patient than for any physiological effect.

Placebo effect – The idea that your brain can convince your body a fake treatment is the real thing—and thus stimulate healing.

Press Ganey Associates – Press Gainey Associates is a South Bend, Indiana–based healthcare company known for developing and distributing patient satisfaction surveys. As of January 2017, its Medical Practice Survey was the most widely used outpatient satisfaction survey in the Unites States.

Psychoneuroimmunology (PNI) – Is the study of the interaction between psychological processes and the nervous and immune systems of the human body. PNI takes an interdisciplinary approach, incorporating psychology, neuroscience, immunology, physiology, genetics, pharmacology, molecular biology, psychiatry, behavioral medicine, infectious diseases, endocrinology, and rheumatology. The main interests of PNI are the interactions between the nervous and immune systems and the relationships between mental processes and health.

Psychopharmacology – Is the study of the use of medications in treating mental disorders. By studying drug-induced changes in mood, thinking, and behavior. The complexity of this field requires continuous study in order to keep current with new advances.

Psycho-Social Neuroimmunology – The study of the influence of psycho-social factors on the immune system and their role for the incidence and progression of cancer and other diseases.

ROI – Return on investment is a ratio between net profit and cost of investment. A high ROI means the investment's gains compare favorably to its cost. As a performance measure, ROI is used to evaluate the efficiency of an investment or to compare the efficiencies of several different investments.

RVU – Relative value units are a measure of value used in the United States Medicare reimbursement formula for physician services. RVUs are a part of the resource-based relative value scale.

Six Sigma – Six Sigma is a set of techniques and tools for process improvement. It was introduced by American engineer Bill Smith while working for Motorola in 1980. Jack Welch made it central to his business strategy at General Electric in 1995.

TEDx Talk – A **TEDx** is a grassroots initiative, created in the spirit of **TED**'s overall mission to research and discover "Ideas worth spreading." The difference between a TED and **TEDx** events are that the former takes more of a global approach while the latter typically focuses on a local community that concentrates on local voices. "Officially, the "x" in **TEDx** stands for an independently organized **TED** event—but it's more of a **TED** multiplied." Fred Lee presented his **TEDx** in 2011 at **TEDx Maastricht** in Maastricht, Netherlands.

TMI – Too Much Information

TQM – Total Quality Management

Yin and Yang – In Ancient Chinese philosophy, yin and yang is a concept of dualism, describing how seemingly opposite or contrary forces may actually be complimentary, interconnected, and interdependent in the natural world, and how they may give rise to each other as they interrelate to one another.

ENDNOTES

CHAPTER 4

[1] Jeffrey Pfeffer and Robert I. Sutton, *The Knowing-Doing Gap: How Smart Companies Turn Knowledge into Action*, (Harvard Business School Press, Jan 2000), Chapter 1.

[2] Amy C. Edmondson, "Strategies for Learning from Failure," (Harvard Business Review, April 2011).

[3] Christopher P. Landrigan, MD, MPH, et al., "Temporal Trends in Rates of Patient Harm Resulting from Medical Care" (*New England Journal of Medicine*, November 25, 2010), 363:2124-2134, DOI: 10.1056/NEJMsa1004404.

[4] Richard M.J. Bohmer, "Fixing Health Care on the Front Lines,"(Harvard Business Review, April 2010).

CHAPTER 5

[5] Hans Selye, "A Syndrome produced by Diverse Nocuous Agents," (Nature, 1936), vol. 138:32.

[6] Walter B. Cannon, MD, CB, *Bodily Changes in Pain, Hunger, Fear and Rage*. (New York: Appleton-Century-Crofts, 1920), p.211.

[7] Hans Selye, "Stress and the general adaptation syndrome," *Br Med J*, no. 1(4667) (1950): 1383-1392. DOI:10.1136/bmj.1.4667.1383.

[8] Selye, "Stress and the general adaptation syndrome," 1383-1392.

[9] Robert M. Sapolsky, *Why Zebras Don't Get Ulcers: An Updated Guide to Stress, Stress-Related Diseases, and Coping*. (New York: W.H. Freeman), 2nd Edition, 1998.

[10] Robert Ader and Nicholas Cohen, "Behaviorally Conditioned Immunosuppression," *Psychosom Med* 37 no. 4, (Jul-Aug 1975), 333-40.

[11] Robert Ader, David L. Felten, and Nicholas Cohen, *Psychoneuroimmunology*, 4th edition, 2 volumes, (Academic Press, 2006), ISBN: 0-12-088576-X.

[12] Phillip T. Marucha, Janice Kiecolt-Glaser, and Mehrdad Favagehi, "Mucosal wound healing is impaired by examination stress," *Psychosomatic Medicine* 60, no. 3 (1998): 362-5.

[13] Gordon D. Schiff, MD, et al., "Ten Principles for More Conservative, Care-Full Diagnosis," *Annals of Intern Medicine* 169, no. 9 (2018): 643–645, DOI: 10.7326/M18-1468.

CHAPTER 6

[14] George L. Engel, "The need for a new medical model: a challenge for biomedicine," *Science* 196, no. 4286 (Apr 1977): 129-36.

[15] Marcus Buckingham and Curt Coffman, *First, Break All the Rules: What the World's Greatest Managers Do Differently*, (New York, NY: Simon & Schuster, 1999).

[16] Ted J. Kaptchuk and Franklin G. Miller, "Placebo Effects in Medicine," *N Engl J Med* 373, no. 1 (Jul 2015): 8-9.

[17] "Putting the placebo effect to work," *Harvard Health Letter*, (Harvard Health Publishing), https://www.health.harvard.edu/mind-and-mood/putting-the-placebo-effect-to-work

[18] Andrea Cipriani, MD, et al., "Comparative efficacy and acceptability of 21 antidepressant drugs for the acute treatment of adults with major depressive disorder: a systematic review and network meta-analysis," *The Lancet* 391, no. 10128 (Feb 21, 2018): 1357-66, accessed April 2020.

[19] Mohammadreza Hojat et al., "Physicians' empathy and clinical outcomes for diabetic patients," *Academic Medicine* 86, no. 3 (March 2011): 359-64.

[20] Stephano Del Canale et al., "The relationship between physician empathy and disease complications: an empirical study of primary care physicians and their diabetic patients in Parma, Italy," *Academic Medicine* 87, no. 9 (Sept 2012): 1243-9.

CHAPTER 7

[21] Stephen Trzeciak and Anthony Mazzarelli, *Compassionomics: The Revolutionary Scientific Evidence that Caring Makes a Difference*, (Fire Starter, 2019).

[22] Beth A. Lown, Julie Rosen, and John Marttila, "An agenda for improving compassionate care: a survey shows about half of patients say such care is missing," *Health Affairs* 30, no. 9 (September 2011): 1772-8.

[23] The Schwartz Center for Compassionate Healthcare, "National Survey Data Presented at the Compassion in Action Conference Show Mixed Reactions on State of Compassion in US Healthcare," News release, June 27, 2017.

[24] Janie Kofford Ford, RN, MS, CFRN, "I'll Take Passion for $1000," *Air Medical Journal Associates* 31, no. 3 (May-Jun 2012):144. DOI: 10.1016/j.amj.2012.03.006.

[25] Francis W. Peabody, MD, "The Care of the Patient" *JAMA* 88, no. 12 (1927): 877-882.

[26] H. Brownell Wheeler, MD, "Healing and Heroism," *N Engl J Med* 322 (1990): 1540-48.

[27] Peter Tyson, "The Hippocratic Oath Today," https://www.pbs.org/wgbh/nova/article/hippocratic-oath-today/, (March 26, 2001), accessed online June 29, 2019.

[28] Peabody, "The Care of the Patient," 877-882.

[29] Mariano E. Menendez, MD, et al., "Physician Empathy as a Driver of Hand Surgery Patient Satisfaction," *Journal of Hand Surgery* 40, no. 9, (2015): 1860-1865.e2.

[30] Aubrey Hill, "Empathy: The First Step to Improving Health Outcomes," *Health Affairs Blog*, February 25, 2014, DOI: 10.1377/hblog20140225.037133

[31] Diane S. Morse, MD, Elizabeth A. Edwardsen, MD, Howard S. Gordon, MD, "Missed opportunities for interval empathy in lung cancer communication," *Arch Intern Med* 168, no. 17, (2008): 1853-1858.

[32] Rick Hanson, PhD, "How Did Humans Become Empathetic?" *Psychology Today*, (Mar 3, 2010), https://www.psychologytoday.com/us/blog/your-wise-brain/201003/how-did-humans-become-empathic

[33] David I. Jeffrey, "Empathy, sympathy and compassion in healthcare: Is there a problem? Is there a difference? Does it matter?" *Journal of the Royal Society of Medicine* 109, no. 12, (2016): 446-452.

[34] Jodi Halpern, MD, PhD, "What is clinical empathy?" *J Gen Intern Med* 18, no. 8, (2003): 670-674.

[35] Helen Riess, "The Impact of Clinical Empathy on Patients and Clinicians: Understanding Empathy's Side Effects," *AJOB Neuroscience* 6, no. 3, (2015): 51-53.

[36] Managed Healthcare Executive, "New C-suite position to watch: Chief Experience Officers," (April 2, 2017) https://www.managedhealthcareexecutive.com/hospitals-providers/new-c-suite-position-watch-chief-experience-officers

[37] Frans Derksen, Jozien Bensing, and Antoine Lagro-Janssen, "Effectiveness of empathy in general practice: a systematic review," *British Journal of General Practice* 63, no. 606, (2013): e76-e84.

[38] Hojat, "Physicians' empathy and clinical outcomes for diabetic patients," 359-64.

[39] David P. Rakel, MD, et al., "Practitioner Empathy and the Duration of the Common Cold," *Fam Med* 41, no. 7, (2009): 494-501.

[40] Ted J. Kaptchuk et al., "Components of placebo effect: randomised controlled trial in patients with irritable bowel syndrome," *BMJ* 336, no. 7651, (2008): 999-1003.

[41] Mohammadreza Hojat, PhD, et al., "Empathy in Medical Education and Patient Care," *Academic Medicine* 76, no. 7, (2001): 669.

[42] Del Canale, "The Relationship Between Physician Empathy and Disease Complications: An Empirical Study of Primary Care Physicians and Their Diabetic Patients in Parma, Italy," 1243-1249.

[43] Debra L. Roter et al., "Effectiveness of interventions to improve patient compliance: a meta-analysis," *Med Care* 36, no. 8, (1998):1131-61.

44 Sandra van Dulmen and Atie van den Brink-Muinen, "Patients' preferences and experiences in handling emotions: A study on communication sequences in primary care medical visits," *Patient Education and Counseling* 55, no. 1 (2004): 149-52.

45 Afaf Girgis and R W. Sanson-Fisher, "Breaking bad news: consensus guidelines for medical practitioners," *J Clin Oncol* 13, no. 9, (1995): 2449-56.

46 Helen Riess et al., "Empathy training for resident physicians: a randomized controlled trial of a neuroscience-informed curriculum," *J Gen Intern Med* 27 no. 10, (2012):1280-6

47 Michael S. Krasner, MD, et al., "Association of an educational program in mindful communication with burnout, empathy, and attitudes among primary care physicians," *JAMA* 302, no. 12, (2009):1284-1293.

48 Tait D. Shanafelt, "Enhancing meaning in work: a prescription for preventing physician burnout and promoting patient-centered care," *JAMA* 302, no. 12 (2009): 1338-1340.

49 Colin P. West, Tait D. Shanafelt, and J.C. Kolars, "Quality of life, burnout, educational debt, and medical knowledge among internal medicine residents," *JAMA* 306, no. 9, (2009): 952-960.

50 Wendy Levinson, Cara S. Lesser, and Ronald M. Epstein, "Developing Physician Communication Skills For Patient-Centered Care," *Health Affairs* 29, no. 7 (2010): 1310-18.

51 Tait D. Shanafelt et al., "Relationship between increased personal well-being and enhanced empathy among internal medicine residents," *J Gen Intern Med* 20, no. 7 (2005):559-64

52 Jodi Halpern, MD, PhD, "Gathering the Patient's Story and Clinical Empathy," *The Permanente Journal* 16, no. 1 (2012):52–54. DOI:10.7812/tpp/11-107

53 Michael S. Krasner, MD, et al., "Association of an educational program in mindful communication with burnout, empathy, and attitudes among primary care physicians," *JAMA* 302, no. 12 (2009): 1284-93.

54 Shanafelt, "Enhancing meaning in work: a prescription for preventing physician burnout and promoting patient-centered care," 1338-40.

55 West, Shanafelt, and Kolars, "Quality of life, burnout, educational debt, and medical knowledge among internal medicine residents," 952-60.

56 Sung Su Kim, Stan Kaplowitz, and Mark V. Johnston, "The Effects of Physician Empathy on Patient Satisfaction and Compliance," *Evaluation & the Health Professions* 27, no. 3 (2004): 237-251.

57 Mohammadreza Hojat et al., "Patient perceptions of physician empathy, satisfaction with physician, interpersonal trust, and compliance," *Int J Med Educ* 1 (2010): 83-87.

[58] Anthony L. Suchman et al., "A model of empathic communication in the medical interview," *JAMA* 277, no. 8 (1997): 678-82.

[59] Hojat, "Physicians' empathy and clinical outcomes for diabetic patients," 359-64.

[60] Suchman et al., "A model of empathic communication in the medical interview," 678-82.

[61] H T. Stelfox et al., "The relation of patient satisfaction with complaints against physicians and malpractice lawsuits," *The American Journal of Medicine* 118, no. 10 (2005): 1126-33.

[62] Halpern, "Gathering the patient's story and clinical empathy," 52-54.

[63] Empathetics, "Why Empathy? More satisfied patients, higher reimbursement, less stress," http://empathetics.com/why-empathy/ accessed April 2020.

[64] United States Census Bureau, "Older People Projected to Outnumber Children for First Time in US History," March 13, 2018, https://www.census.gov/newsroom/press-releases/2018/cb18-41-population-projections.html

[65] Kevin J. Kelley, PhD, and Mary F. Kelley, MSN, RN, CRNP, "Teaching Empathy and Other Compassion-Based Communication Skills," *Journal for Nurses in Professional Development* 29, no. 6 (2013): 321-24.

[66] Riess et al., "Empathy Training for Resident Physicians: A Randomized Controlled Trial of a Neuroscience-Informed Curriculum," 1280.

[67] Helen Riess, MD, and Gordon Kraft-Todd, "E.M.P.A.T.H.Y.:A Tool to Enhance Nonverbal Communication Between Clinicians and Their Patients," *Acad Med* 89, no. 8 (2014): 1108-12.

[68] David Lawrence, MD, *From Chaos to Care: The Promise of Team-Based Medicine*: Da Capo Lifelong Books (2003), 69-71.

CHAPTER 8

[69] Carmine Gallo, *The Storyteller's Secret: From TED Speakers to Business Legends, Why Some Ideas Catch On and Others Don't*: St Martin's Press (2017)

[70] Rita Charon, MD, PhD, "Narrative medicine: form, function, and ethics," *Ann Intern Med* 134, no. 1 (2001): 83-87.

[71] Rita Charon, MD, PhD, "Narrative Medicine: A Model for Empathy, Reflection, Profession, and Trust," *JAMA* 286, no. 15 (2001): 1897-1902.

[72] David B. Morris, *Illness and Culture in the Postmodern Age* (Berkeley: University of California Press, 2000).

[73] Melvin Konner, MD, *Medicine at the Crossroads: The Crisis in Health Care* (New York, NY: Pantheon Books, 1993).

[74] Engel, "The need for a new medical model: a challenge for biomedicine," 129-136.

[75] Christine Laine, MD, MPH, and Frank Davidoff, MD, "Patient-centered medicine: a professional evolution," *JAMA* 275, no. 2 (1996):152-156.

[76] Charon, "Narrative Medicine: A Model for Empathy, Reflection, Profession, and Trust," 1897-1902.

[77] Ben Kesling, "To Improve Care, Veterans Affairs Asks Patients Their Life Stories," https://www.wsj.com/articles/to-improve-care-veterans-affairs-asks-patients-their-life-stories-11562146202, Published July 2, 2019, Accessed July 5, 2019.

[78] Gallo, *The Storyteller's Secret: From TED Speakers to Business Legends, Why Some Ideas Catch On and Others Don't*.

[79] Jerome Groopman, MD, *How Doctors Think* (Houghton Mifflin Harcourt, 2008), email permission received.

CHAPTER 9

[80] Quint Studer, *Hardwiring Excellence: Purpose, Worthwhile Work, Making a Difference* (Fire Starter Publishing: Studer Group, 2003).

[81] Jozien M. Bensing, W. Verheul, and A.M. Van Dulmen, "Patient anxiety in the medical encounter: a study of verbal and nonverbal communication in general practice," *Health Education* 108, no. 5 (2008): 373-83.

[82] Linda A. Fogarty et al., "Can 40 Seconds of Compassion Reduce Patient Anxiety?" *Journal of Clinical Oncology* 17, no. 1 (1999): 371-79

[83] Trzeciak, *Compassionomics: The Revolutionary Scientific Evidence that Caring Makes a Difference*, 257.

[84] Thomas Joiner, *Why People Die by Suicide* (Cambridge: Harvard University Press, 2007).

[85] Leeza Gibbons et.al., *Take Your Oxygen First: Protecting Your Health and Happiness While Caring for a Loved One with Memory Loss* (LaChance Publishing, 2009).

[86] Helen Wilkinson et al., "Examining the Relationship between Burnout and Empathy in Healthcare Professionals: A Systematic Review," *Burnout Research* 6, (September 2017): 18-29.

[87] Matthew R. Thomas et al., "How Do Distress and Well-being Relate to Medical Student Empathy? A Multicenter Study," *Journal of General Internal Medicine* 22, no 2 (2007): 177-83.

[88] Trzeciak, *Compassionomics: The Revolutionary Scientific Evidence that Caring Makes a Difference*, 295.

[89] Hui-Ching Weng et al., "Doctor's Emotional Intelligence and the Patient-Doctor Relationship," *Medical Education* 42, no. 7 (2008): 703-11.

[90] "Doctors' Interpersonal Skills Are Valued More Than Training," *The Wall Street Journal* Online, https://www.wsj.com/articles/SB109630288893728881; article updated Sept 28, 2004, accessed April 2020.

[91] Wilkinson, "Examining the Relationship between Burnout and Empathy in Healthcare Professionals: A Systematic Review," 18-29.

[92] Olga Klimecki and Tania Singer, "Empathic distress fatigue rather than compassion fatigue? Integrating findings from empathy research in psychology and social neuroscience," Chapter 28 in *Pathological Altruism* (New York, NY: Oxford University Press, 2011): 368-83.

[93] Riess et al., "Empathy training for resident physicians: a randomized controlled trial of a neuroscience-informed curriculum," 1280-86

[94] Donald M. Berwick, Thomas W. Nolan, and John Whittington, "The Triple Aim: Care, Health, and Cost," *Health Affairs* 27, no. 3 (2008): 759-69.

[95] Hojat, "Physicians' empathy and clinical outcomes for diabetic patients," 359-64.

[96] Megha Bansal et al., "Impact of Reducing Glycated Hemoglobin on Healthcare Costs Among a Population with Uncontrolled Diabetes," *Appl Health Econ Health Policy*, 16, no. 5 (2018): 675-84.

[97] Cleveland Clinic Orthopaedic Arthroplasty, "The Association Between Readmission and Patient Experience in a Total Hip Arthroplasty Population," *The Journal of Arthroplasty* 33, no. 6 (2017).

[98] Jill Maben et al., "A realist informed mixed-methods evaluation of Schwartz Center Rounds® in England," *Southampton (UK): NIHR Journals Library* (Nov 2018).

[99] Katie Owens et al., "The Imperative of Culture: a quantitative analysis of the impact of culture on workforce engagement, patient experience, physician engagement, value-based purchasing, and turnover," *Journal of Healthcare Leadership* 2017, no 9, (2017): 26.

[100] Owens et al., "The Imperative of Culture: a quantitative analysis of the impact of culture on workforce engagement, patient experience, physician engagement, value-based purchasing, and turnover," 25-31.

[101] Sigal G. Barsade and Olivia A. O'Neill, "What's Love Got to Do With It? A Longitudinal Study of the Culture of Companionate Love and Employee and Client Outcomes in a Long-term Care Setting," *Administrative Science Quarterly* 59, no. 4 (2014): 551-98.

CHAPTER 10

[102] Simon Sinek, *Start with Why: How Great Leaders Inspire Everyone to Take Action* (Portfolio Publishing, 2009).

[103] Christina Maslach and Michael P. Leiter, "Understanding the burnout experience: recent research and its implications for psychiatry," *World Psychiatry* 15, no. 2 (2016): 103-111.

[104] Audrey Lyndon, PhD, "Perspectives on Safety: Burnout Among Health Professionals and Its Effect on Patient Safety," *PS Net: Agency for Healthcare Research and Quality* (Jan 2015).

[105] Louise H. Hall et al., "Healthcare Staff Wellbeing, Burnout, and Patient Safety: A Systematic Review," PLoS ONE 11, no. 7 (2016): e0159015

[106] Alexandra Robbins, "The Problem With Satisfied Patients: A misguided attempt to improve healthcare has led some hospitals to focus on making people happy, rather than making them well," (Apr 17, 2015).

[107] Brian Colosi, BA, MBA, SPHR—President, "2016 National Healthcare Retention & RN Staffing Report," *NSI Nursing Solutions Inc.* (March 2016).

[108] Bridget Duffy, MD, "For Better Outcomes, Add One Part Joy," *Health IT Outcomes* (Guest Column—Nov 17, 2017).

[109] About Us page of The Schwartz Center for Compassionate Healthcare website, accessed April 2020, https://www.theschwartzcenter.org/about/who-we-are.

HEARTWIRING TOOLKIT

[110] Smart Goals Guide website, accessed April 12, 2020, https://www.smart-goals-guide.com.

[111] Loren Eiseley, *The Star Thrower* (Houghton Mifflin Harcourt Publishing Company, 1978).

[112] John Parrington, PhD, "Working together is part of what makes us human," *Socialist Worker* 2427 (Oct 2014).